Thank you to the members of these ISNA Regions
for their financial support of this publication.

North Region

Southwest Region

West Region

West Central Region

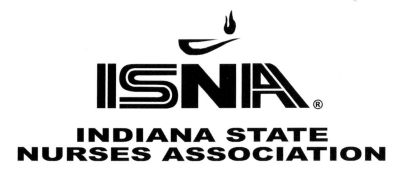

ISNA®

**INDIANA STATE
NURSES ASSOCIATION**

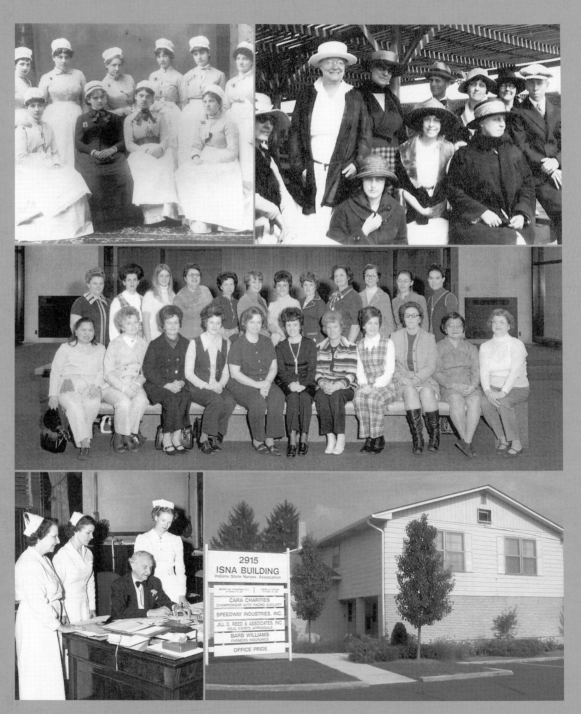

THE
DONNING COMPANY
PUBLISHERS

Advocacy and Action

100 Years of Indiana Nursing and the
Indiana State Nurses Association

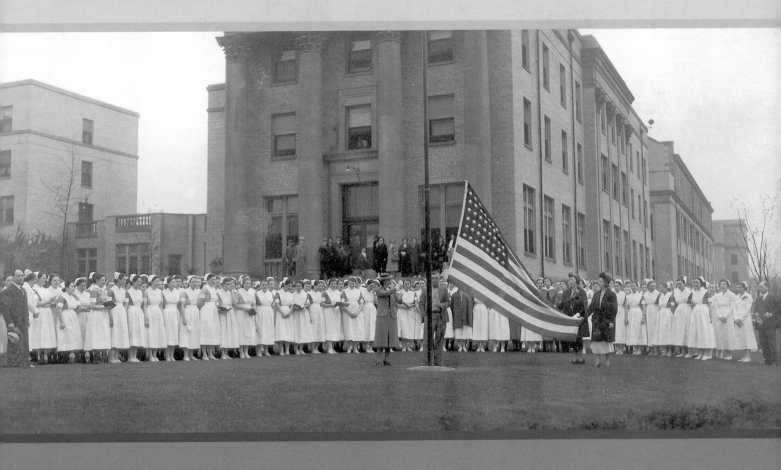

Edited by
Marjorie Lentz Porter, Ed.D., R.N.
Barbra Mann Wall, Ph.D., R.N.

COVER (clockwise from top left):

Nurses assisting in surgery at City Hospital (Indianapolis) in 1887. (ISNA Collection M0380, Indiana Historical Society)

A panel at the Inter-Group Relations Institute, at Indiana University's Student Union in Bloomington, in February 1957. Pictured (L to R) are Dean Long, Evansville College; Sister Miriam Dolores, Anderson; Pauline Eans, Indianapolis General; Howard Lytle, Goodwill Industries, Indianapolis; Father Raymond Bosler, Indiana Catholic and Record, Indianapolis; Dr. Leon Levi, M.D., Indianapolis; Edmund Shea, Indiana University Hospitals, Indianapolis. (ISNA Collection M0380, Indiana Historical Society)

Prescriptive authority becomes law: ISNA took a leading role in working with legislators and developing the language of Indiana's law that granted prescriptive authority to advanced-practice nurses. ISNA members attend the ceremony where Governor Evan Bayh signed the measure into law in 1993. Front row: Dr. Jon C. Bailey, Indiana health commissioner, and Governor Bayh. Back row: Kari Berron; Naomi Patchin, ISNA executive director; Esther Acree, chair, Council of Nurses in Advanced Practice; and A. Louise Hart, ISNA president.

Indianapolis was the site for the 1908 ISNA Annual Meeting. While many of the members are not identified, the known delegates are: First row: 1. E. Gertrude Fournier, first president; 2. Anna Rein; 3. Mae Currie; 4. Edna Humphrey; 5. Mary Sollers; 6. Minnie Prange. Second row: 1. Frances Teague; 2. Frances Ott; 4. Florence Martin; 9. Stella Cotton; 14. May Rutan Baylor; 15. Mae Gentry. Third row: 2. Jeanette Miller; 7. Cora Nifer; 8. Elizabeth Johnson; 13. Cora Williams; 16. Miss Evans; 17. Ida McCaslin. (ISNA Archives)

ISNA representatives to the 1958 American Nurses Association convention in Atlantic City, New Jersey. (L to R) Mary Ann Robertson, Kathryn Lawson, Jane Lee Jenkins, Thelma Sanders, Norma Mattingly, Louise Phillabaum, Norma Jean Watkins, Pearl Long, and Wilma Green. (ISNA Collection M0380, Indiana Historical Society)

Indiana University School of Nursing students, from the class of 1929, in an advertisement promoting subscriptions to The American Journal of Nursing. The Lamp, October 1949. (ISNA Collection M0380, Indiana Historical Society)

Copyright © 2003 by Indiana State Nurses Association.
Ernest C. Klein, Jr., R.N., CAE, Executive Director

The Donning Company Publishers
184 Business Park Drive, Suite 206
Virginia Beach, VA 23452

Steve Mull, General Manager
Barbara B. Buchanan, Office Manager
Ed Williams, Project Director
Cindy Smith, Project Research Coordinator
Kathleen Sheridan, Editor
Jeremy Gray, Graphic Designer
Daniel Carr, Imaging Artist
Mary Ellen Wheeler, Proofreader/Editorial Assistant
Scott Rule, Director of Marketing
Travis Gallup, Marketing Coordinator

Library of Congress Cataloging-in-Publication Data

Advocacy and action : 100 years of Indiana Nursing and the Indiana State Nurses Association / edited by Marjorie Lentz Porter, Barbra Mann Wall.
    p. cm.
Includes bibliographical references and index.
  ISBN 1-57864-232-9
  1. Nursing--Indiana--History. I. Porter, Marjorie Lentz. II. Wall, Barbra Mann.
  RT5.I6A385 2003
  610.73'06'0772--dc22

                                      2003021401

Printed in the United States of America

Table of Contents

Foreword

The Indiana State Nurses Association celebrates its one hundredth anniversary in 2003. Founded in Fort Wayne as one of the first professional nurse associations in the United States, the ISNA continues to be the voice for Indiana's registered nurses. This past century was the most successful and turbulent in modern world history. You need look no further than the health care field to see this extraordinary evolution.

From its inception, the ISNA has stressed the educational preparation and professional excellence of the registered nurse. These values have served our members well as their scope of practice has expanded through the years. Compared with previous generations, today's nurse has more autonomy in the practice of nursing, which requires expanded skills and greater knowledge. The ISNA works with the state's schools of nursing—their deans, directors and educators—and the Indiana State Board of Nursing to maintain and promote educational standards for nurses.

Government relations are also a key to the ISNA's success. Our members' opinions and feedback are routinely sought by elected leaders and government officials. Even during the first half of the 1900s, when women were rarely at the public policy table, the ISNA's female leadership forged relationships, built coalitions, and regularly developed and established health care rules and regulations. We continue to participate in the legislative process and lend our voice to ensure the interests of professional nurses are heard and protected.

The ISNA encourages and promotes a healthy workplace. Nurses face threats each day to their person—including needle sticks, latex allergies, repetitive back injuries, and workplace violence. Also, time is becoming increasingly scarce as the nurse shortage and mandatory overtime continue to be a drain on individuals and the profession. The association has joined with groups to find solutions to these issues and is partnering with individual facilities and members to improve working conditions.

Dedicated nurses continue to be the backbone of the health care system, and the public continues to rate our profession as one of the most trusted. I would like to thank the members of the history book committee whose many hours of research and writing have made this publication possible. Your dedication and hard work will be enjoyed by generations to come. I hope you enjoy reading about the history of the ISNA and the role the association continues to play in shaping the course of nursing in Indiana.

Sandra Fights, President
Indiana State Nurses Association

Preface

This publication is a history of the Indiana State Nurses Association in commemoration of its centennial year. It tells a story not only of the association but also of nursing in Indiana, including the events, persons, and forces that have shaped it. The book is not meant to be an all-inclusive history, as the limitations of space and time made it impossible to detail all events and persons who were a part of this story.

The authors have constructed the book largely from primary source material and have followed a chronological and topical organization. Within this framework, we have illustrated the ISNA's response to major events such as wars and depressions, and we have integrated issues of gender, race, economics, and community history as the sources have allowed. Several themes weave throughout the chapters, including collaboration, advocacy, service, and leadership. Of interest in the early years is the contrast between traditional ideas about gender and the very real accomplishments women made. In an era when women were so subordinate that they could not even vote, the founding members of the association successfully promoted and acquired registered nurse licensure. From helping nurses who were unemployed in the 1930s to political action in the 1990s, the ISNA has consistently effected change for the betterment of the public and the nursing profession.

The ISNA has always worked closely with the Indiana State Board of Nursing. The board is presently under the auspices of the Bureau of Health Professions, but in the early years, it was variously known as the State Board of Examination and Registration for Nurses and the State Board of Nurses' Registration and Nursing Education. The authors have used the terms State Board and Board of Nursing interchangeably to reflect this organization.

Today, the ISNA continues to represent Indiana nurses with professionalism and dedication. In the words of former Executive Director Naomi Patchin, "Indiana may not always be first, but what we do, we do well."

The development, writing, and editing of this book have been the collective effort of many dedicated individuals. We would like to thank the ISNA staff—Ernest Klein, Gary Abell, Barbara Carrico, and Sara Denny—for their valuable contributions of time, space, and expertise. We thank Brenda Lyon, Ann Marriner-Tomey, Sharon Isaac, Naomi Patchin, and Ernest Klein for granting personal interviews. Working behind the scenes was Juanita Laidig, who provided valuable information and personal encouragement. Appreciation is also extended to the University of Indianapolis and Purdue University, who gave the editors release time and monetary support. The Indiana Historical Society and Wishard Hospital School of Nursing History Museum are acknowledged for supplying rich sources of data and photographs from their valuable collections. Approval for this research was granted through the respective committees for the protection of human subjects at the University of Indianapolis and Purdue University.

To all those who were involved, we are grateful. Mostly, we appreciate having the privilege of learning about the extraordinary nurses who make up this important story.

Marjorie Lentz Porter
Barbra Mann Wall

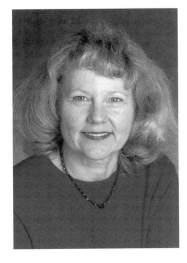

Marjorie Lentz Porter, Ed.D., R.N., is an Associate Professor at University of Indianapolis School of Nursing.

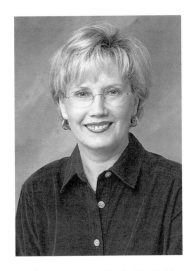

Barbra Mann Wall, Ph.D., R.N., is an Assistant Professor at Purdue University School of Nursing.

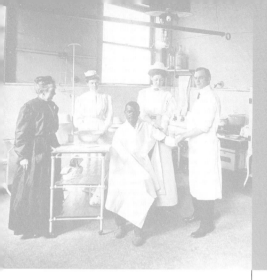

Chapter 1

History of Nursing in Indiana
1860-1900

Kathleen Pickrell, M.S.N., R.N., and Karla Backer, Ph.D., R.N.

Monument to Eliza George, Fort Wayne, Indiana (Photo courtesy of Kathleen Pickrell, M.S.N., R.N.)

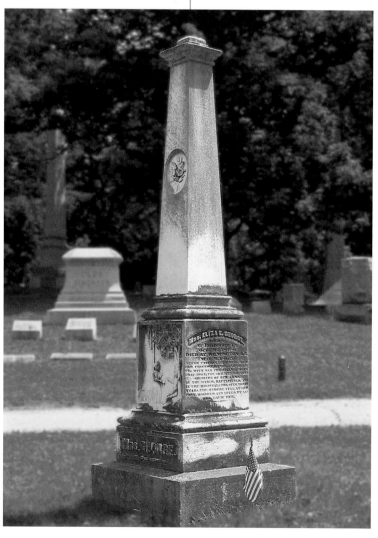

In 1863 during the peak of the Civil War, fifty-five-year-old Eliza George left her home in Fort Wayne, Indiana, as a representative of the Indiana Sanitary Commission. Formed in 1862 by Governor Oliver P. Morton, the Indiana Sanitary Commission provided supplies, land and water transportation services, and nursing and medical care to thousands of Hoosier soldiers. As a nurse, Mrs. George helped establish hospitals in Pulaski, Tennessee, and Corinth, Mississippi. She cared for the wounded during General Sherman's Georgia campaign, and she worked with the ambulance service to transport wounded soldiers from battlefields in Georgia and Tennessee. Mrs. George served behind the battle lines, cooking and helping to care for thousands of men. Sometimes she was in the direct line of fire. When the war ended, she continued her work by nursing former prisoners of war in Wilmington, North Carolina. While there, she contracted typhoid fever, and due to her age and the exertions of the previous two years, she was unable to fight the infection. Governor Morton had sent Dr. William Henry Wishard to look after Indiana veterans as far south as Wilmington. While there, Dr. Wishard cared for Mrs. George, but in spite of his efforts, she died. He personally accompanied her body back to Fort Wayne. The Indiana Sanitary Commission recognized her service by erecting a monument to her in that city.[1]

In the years before the Civil War, most women provided nursing care in the home as part of their domestic duties, but it was limited to family members or friends. There were a few "natural born" or "professed" nurses who cared for non family members to provide incomes for themselves. For women in isolated areas, the "family doctor book" was one of the few sources of medical information available.[2] Some of the earliest nurses in Indiana were Catholic sisters, who had extensive experience in nursing people outside the home environment. When a woman joined a religious order, she intentionally undertook the role of caretaker to persons beyond the family circle.

The environment of the early settlers contributed to unhealthy living conditions and exposed them to disease and infection. Swampy, underwater woodlands, wet river bottoms, and deep forests that bred mosquitoes and houseflies caused diseases such as malaria and typhoid fever.[3] Many early settlers lived in open cabins or tents with diets that consisted mainly of game and fish. Others raised wheat, corn, beef, and pork. Sanitation and good hygiene were nonexistent.[4] Cholera thrived in such conditions and was the cause of the most severe epidemics of the nineteenth century. It struck Indiana in 1833 and again in 1848. Interest in public health paralleled outbreaks of disease. In 1830, for example, smallpox broke out in the Indianapolis area, and although it did not become an epidemic as predicted, residents were terrified, called a public meeting, and created a Board of Health. The Board recommended building a hospital, but public interest declined once the epidemic subsided.[5]

Settlers who lived in remote areas were less likely to contract infections as a result of their isolation, but infectious diseases were common in the larger settlements. In addition to cholera, the most devastating illnesses were typhoid and malarial fevers, pneumonia, tuberculosis, and bronchitis. Among children, diseases such as croup and cholera infantum caused the highest mortality rates.[6] Few who practiced medicine were formally educated. Many treatments and procedures harmed more persons than they helped or cured.

When the population of Indianapolis swelled to 20,000 in 1854, the hospital issue reemerged. After another smallpox outbreak, the City Council approved hospital construction. The hospital, begun in 1855 and completed four years later, proved to be a costly and controversial undertaking. Construction was slow due to lack of funding, and citizens were divided in their support. Some saw the hospital as an asset to a growing city; others questioned the need for such an expensive, useless undertaking.[7]

The outbreak of the Civil War became the catalyst for those in favor of keeping the hospital. Camp Morton, located in the state fairgrounds in Indianapolis, became a central location for Indiana volunteers to assemble and train. Civil War army camps were notoriously unhealthy environments. Men tossed refuse and garbage wherever they wished, and some refused to use the latrines. Camps, then, became breeding sites for disease. Throughout the four-year conflict, more casualties resulted from disease than from battle. On average, soldiers were ill from disease more than twice each year, and death rates exceeded fifty-three per thousand.[8] At the same time, the state of medical knowledge was rudimentary. Historian James M. McPherson writes, "The Civil War was fought at the end of the medical Middle Ages."[9] The revolution of the germ theory came too late to help these soldiers.

At the beginning of the war, the medical departments of both the Union and Confederate armies had to assemble whole new medical systems, and early efforts at care were often disorganized. Hospitals typically were wooden buildings or old hotels with dirty walls and floors. Union soldiers complained of the unsanitary hospital conditions and the fact that they had few good nurses. At the start of the war, various women's groups were eager to extend their domestic skills and volunteered as nurses. Many served under reformer Dorothea Dix, who had been named "Superintendent of Female Nurses" for the Army in 1861. Others worked with agencies such as the U.S. Sanitary Commission. Catholic sisters did not volunteer individually as nurses; rather, medical and military authorities or priests specifically requested them. By the end of the war, nearly 10,000 women had served as nurses either with the Army or with the Sanitary Commission. Of these, 617 were nuns.[10]

"I Go to Indianapolis to See about…the Hospital"

One of the earliest sites for organized delivery of nursing care during the Civil War was the City Hospital in Indianapolis, which Governor Morton offered as a military hospital to the United States government in 1861. The editor of the local newspaper noted that the hospital had been abandoned and "lewd women and vagabond men [had] turned it into a monstrous brothel."[11] But an outbreak of measles in the nearby camp necessitated its use once again as a hospital. Thus the facility, which had created so much controversy in previous years, was finally put to use as a medical unit. At Governor Morton's request, nuns from the Sisters of Providence of Saint-Mary-of-the-Woods, Indiana, arrived to provide the nursing care. In May 1861 Mother Mary Cecelia, superior general of the Sisters of Providence, wrote in her diary:

> *I go to Indianapolis to see about the offer we have to take care of the soldiers in the hospital. The hospital is put under our charge May 17th. The wretched condition of the soldiers is such that the authorities are most anxious to see the Sisters come to take care of the sick. Three Sisters are put in charge of the City Hospital.*[12]

Mother Mary Cecelia chose Sister Athanasius Fogarty to lead the group of sisters, and they worked free of charge. One historian of the congregation noted that the nuns found the hospital in "a state of incredible disorder and filth."[13] The sisters took charge of the nursing, cooking, cleaning, washing, and general housekeeping, with help from male and female attendants. Within a month's time, the *Indianapolis Daily Journal* noted, "[I]t is as complete in its arrangement, clean, well-ventilated, well-provided, and comfortable as any hospital in the country."[14] By March 1863, 5,500 Union soldiers had received treatment, with only 213 deaths, a significantly low mortality rate for that time.[15] The Sisters of Providence also cared for sick soldiers in Vincennes.

Duties of the Civil War nurse can be seen in light of newspaper reports about the military hospital in Indianapolis. The day began at 5:00 a.m. Nurses busied themselves with cleaning spittoons, washing patients' faces and arms, sweeping the wards, dressing wounds, and distributing meals. After breakfast they changed beds and, three times a week, gave the wards a general scrubbing. Throughout the day they distributed beef tea, milk punch, medicines, and other meals, according to directions placed at the head of each bed. During the night they gave more medicines and kept the bandages wet, consistent with the practice of the day.[16]

The Sisters of the Holy Cross from Notre Dame, Indiana, also answered an appeal for Civil War nurses. On 21 October 1861 Governor Morton requested twelve nuns to care for the sick and injured in the Union Army. Mother Angela Gillespie and five other sisters immediately volunteered and left the next morning for Cairo, Illinois. Upon their arrival three days later, they met General Ulysses S. Grant, who sent them to the regimental hospitals of General Lew Wallace's brigade in Paducah, Kentucky. Eventually, nearly eighty Holy Cross Sisters nursed the sick and wounded primarily in Illinois, Missouri, Kentucky, and Tennessee. They also served on the hospital ship *Red Rover*, and for their services there, the Navy has proclaimed them the "first Navy nurses."[17]

In addition to providing nursing care, other women organized aid societies that contributed clothing, blankets, and bedding, and they prepared hospital supplies.[18] They also raised funds to help families of soldiers in the field. Women took a decisive role in the formation of the U.S. Sanitary Commission in 1861. It investigated military hospitals, procured qualified physicians, ran hospital ships, obtained supplies, and developed ambulance services. It also employed women nurses, including Protestant women of the middle and upper classes, African American women, working-class women, and Catholic nuns.[19] The first major test of its goals came after the Battle of Fort Donelson, Tennessee, on 15 and 16 February 1862. Union casualty estimates exceeded 17,000; Indiana casualties alone were greater than 1,000. Many of the wounded froze to death from exposure to the elements. Indianapolis citizens arranged for women to care for the Indiana soldiers there; however, military authorities did not allow them to do so. Instead, after the battle, hospital ships carried the soldiers to other military hospitals where many were nursed by the Sisters of Providence in Vincennes and by Lois Dennett and Harriet Reese Colfax (from Michigan City) in St. Louis City Hospital. Mrs. Colfax also nursed the wounded after the Battle of Shiloh (Tennessee), as did the Sisters of the Holy Cross.[20]

Governor Morton took an aggressive role in organizing help for Indiana soldiers. Through the Indiana Sanitary Commission, the state became one of the most active in the West in providing a well-conducted and systematic organization of care. Within the state, Indiana women nursed in hospital centers at Indianapolis, Jeffersonville, and Evansville. They worked on hospital ships to transport wounded Indiana soldiers after the Vicksburg battle as they returned to northern hospitals. Many Indiana women followed Eliza George's example and traveled to several different facilities. They also held sanitary fairs that supplied materials and goods to troops in the field and in hospitals. In all, approximately 250 nurses served through the Indiana Sanitary Commission. On average, there were about fifty women nurses in the field after 1863.

Women who served in the military hospitals did not have formal training. Indeed, few nurse training schools existed in the United States prior to the Civil War. Those who volunteered often saw nursing as an extension of their mothering and housekeeping roles. Many upper- and middle-class women nurses, for example, asserted that their life experiences in managing households rendered them highly qualified to administer hospitals and nurse the sick and injured.

Women in religious orders, such as the Sisters of Providence and the Sisters of the Holy Cross, learned nursing skills through their life experiences with the poor and needy. Initially, convalescing soldiers worked as nurses, and many surgeons opposed the introduction of women into this role. Dorothea Dix selected her nurses by age (thirty-five years or older), plain-looking appearance, and good reputation, but many physicians criticized the women for being meddlesome.[21] To some doctors, Catholic sisters' traditions of obedience, discipline, and selflessness made them preferable because they were perceived to be less likely to question physicians' orders.[22]

By the war's end, Indiana women had earned the respect of the soldiers and the men in the Sanitary Commission. Its president, William Hannaman, commended Eliza George and the other nurses in his final report to the governor.[23] Their nursing during the Civil War was a critical event in advancing the status of women economically and professionally. They were central players during the war, as they worked alongside doctors and others to set standards for nursing wherever they went. The Civil War became an opportunity for women to improve their image as nurses and to contribute to the development of modern nursing in the United States. Influenced by their wartime work, they developed a nursing model that stressed the importance of maintaining physical and moral cleanliness, order, and discipline.[24]

Separating the Trained from the Untrained

Nursing leaders' crusade to separate the trained from the untrained nurse began in the three decades following the Civil War. In 1873 the first nurse training school based on Florence Nightingale's model opened at Bellevue Hospital in New York. Others soon followed in New Haven and Boston, but there were no such schools in Indiana until 1883. Nurse training schools grew as the general hospital movement accelerated from 1876 to 1900. In Indiana, hospitals opened across the state, bringing a need for skilled nurses who could not only care for the sick but also manage the hospitals. As the supply of nurses was inadequate to meet the needs, some hospitals used nurses prepared in the eastern schools, and others imported nurses from abroad.[25]

The military hospital in Indianapolis operated until the end of the war. In 1865 the Sisters of Providence used the site as St. John's Home for Invalids to care for sick veterans. Then in 1866 City Hospital was reestablished as a municipal institution with a bed capacity of fifty.[26] During the 1860s, most nursing care was unorganized, especially in large city hospitals such as the one in Indianapolis, although some nurses did develop ability for it. One history of City Hospital describes a man and woman who cared for the patients:

> *She was a middle-aged woman who has acquired some experience in nursing one way or another; and as nurses went in those days, she was a "very fair nurse." The male nurse had no previous experience or training, and Dr. Wishard was compelled to terminate his employment because of his personal endeavors to diminish the supply of alcohol in the hospital.*[27]

Convalescents often helped the nurse in caring for the patients. Doctors placed prescribed medications at the bedside with the expectation that patients would take the required dosage at the correct times.[28]

Indiana did not escape the nationwide economic panic in 1873. The poor in Indianapolis were able to obtain free outpatient medical care through the City Dispensary and the Bobbs Free Dispensary, the latter given to the city by Dr. John Bobbs upon his death.[29] Other cities turned to religious orders of women to care for the poor. The Poor Sisters of St. Francis Seraph of Perpetual Adoration came to Lafayette from Germany and established St. Elizabeth Hospital in 1876. With an initial bed capacity of nineteen, the sisters cared for the ill. In 1882 they established St. Anthony's in Terre Haute with a bed capacity of eighteen, and nuns from St. Elizabeth's in Lafayette came to work as nurses. They founded St. Margaret's Hospital in Hammond in 1898. The Daughters of Charity founded St. Vincent's Hospital in Indianapolis in 1881 with a bed capacity of twenty-five. St. Joseph's Hospital in South Bend opened in 1882 under the auspices of the Sisters of the Holy Cross. They expanded their hospital mission to Anderson, where they established St. John Hickey's Memorial Hospital in 1894. In each of these facilities, the nuns served as nurses with a sister-superior as administrator. St. Vincent's supplemented the sisters with nurses from the East who had attended a professional school of nursing.[30]

Other hospitals used Protestant nurses. Fort Wayne City Hospital opened in 1878 and eventually became Hope Hospital.[31] Protestant Deaconess Hospital in Evansville was founded in 1892 with a bed capacity of nineteen. The nurses came from Christ's Hospital in Cincinnati, Ohio, and Drexel Home Hospital in Philadelphia. Union Hospital in Terre Haute, established in 1892, had a bed capacity of eighteen. For the first four years, the facility used inexperienced workers to provide nursing care, but two Deaconess sisters from Cincinnati's Bethesda Hospital came in 1896. Women and men from the Methodist Church founded Memorial Hospital in South Bend in 1893 with an initial bed capacity of twelve.[32]

Nurses from Union Hospital (Terre Haute) in 1900 (ISNA Collection M0380, Indiana Historical Society)

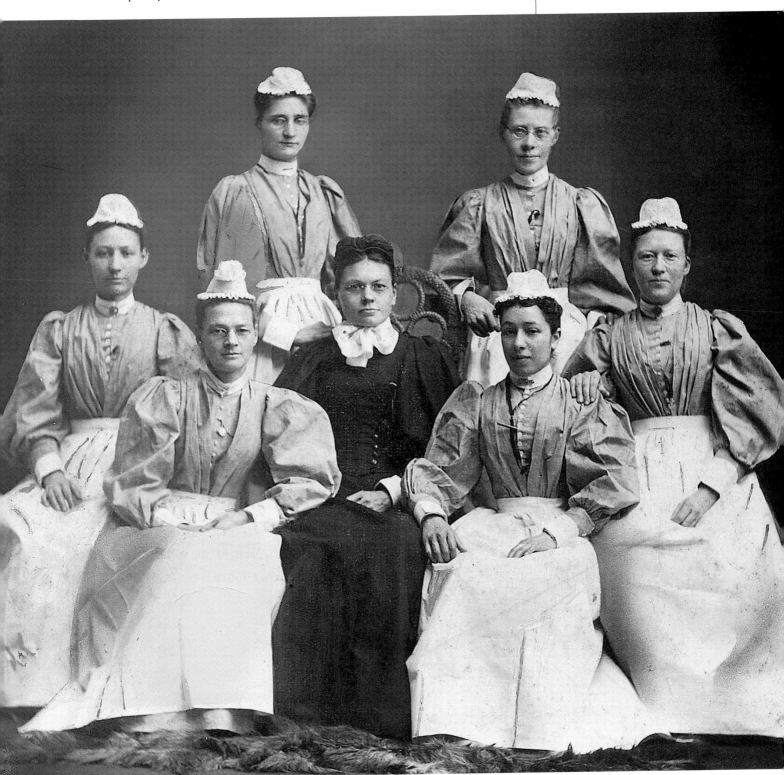

The trend in these early years was to have one nurse in charge of the nursing services. The nurses' functions varied depending on the hospital. Much related to the patients' personal hygiene, namely giving baths to those too ill to care for themselves. Housekeeping responsibilities took up a great amount of time, such as doing the daily laundry with a washtub and board after heating the water on a stove; ironing with a hand iron; mending clothes; and scrubbing, cleaning, and dusting. Nurses also prepared and served the meals. At St. John Hickey's Memorial Hospital in Anderson, the sister-nurses cared for the cows and chickens, which they used to provide milk and eggs for the patients.[33]

As nursing evolved from a service to a trained practice, knowledge of disease prevention, discipline, and organization came to be important qualities of the nurse.[34] In 1883 Indianapolis physician E. F. Hodges wrote to the editor of the *Indianapolis Journal* regarding the need for trained nurses. He was concerned about the practice of unskilled individuals caring for the sick. Implying social distinctions between trained and untrained nurses, he noted that patients had been cared for "by a class of persons for the most part incompetent to obtain a living in any other calling…whose experience merely confirms them in super-stitious reliance upon unusual and often dangerous measures…." He also linked the unskilled nurse with the spread of infection: "With time-honored dread of scarlatina and typhoid fever, we find her going cheerfully from one case of puer-peral fever to another, in the full consciousness of duty done." By contrast, the nursing profession "is recruited from a superior class of young women." Using an argument prescient of one nurses would still be using 120 years later, he con-cluded that intelligent and able trained nurses were due "respect and well-paid employment."[35]

The Beginning of Professional Nurse Training in Indiana

Dr. William Niles Wishard was instrumental in the founding of the first nurse training school in Indiana. He had become superintendent of City Hospital in Indianapolis in 1879 after graduation from Indiana Medical College and Cincinnati's Miami Medical College. In 1883 women of the Flower Mission invited him to their meeting so they could share their idea of a training school for nurses. After establishing the charity in 1876, these prominent women regu-larly took flowers to the sick and poor in their homes and in the hospital, and they saw a ready need for trained nurses. At the 1883 meeting, Dr. Wishard

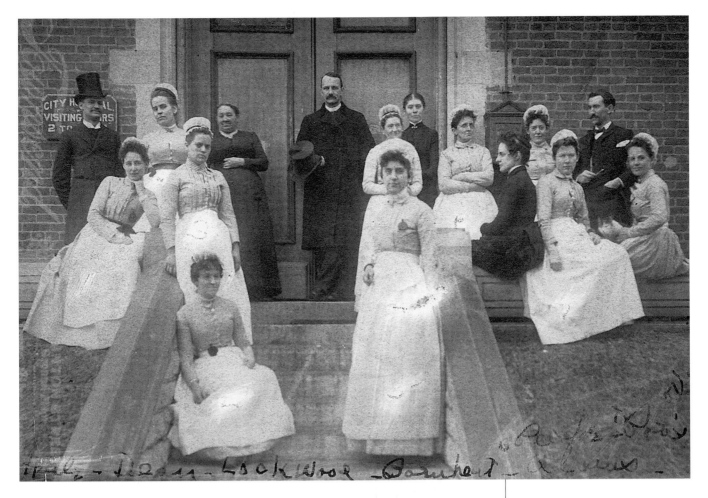

agreed to assist the women in forming a nursing school, and their efforts were successful with the opening of the first Training School for Nurses in Indiana in 1883. This school was only the second program of nursing west of the Allegheny Mountains.[36]

On 1 September 1883 the training school opened in Indianapolis under the supervision of the Flower Mission and in connection with City Hospital. Adele Traver was the first superintendent. As such, she was responsible for training the students and ensuring their proper conduct and comfort. Miss Traver and her two assistants, Miss Richard and Miss Crosby, were Bellevue Hospital graduates. City Hospital paid them $900 a year. They wore black uniforms and white caps, which separated them from the students who wore blue-and-white-striped uniforms with a white apron and cap.[37] Later, each training school established a uniform and cap that became its distinguishing mark. Due to illness, Miss Traver resigned after a year, and Abbie Hunt (later Mrs. Peter Bryce) became superintendent for the next three years. Margaret Iddings was the first student to be admitted to the training school.[38]

Dr. Wishard (center with hat) posed with nurses in front of City Hospital (Indianapolis) in 1887. (ISNA Collection M0380, Indiana Historical Society)

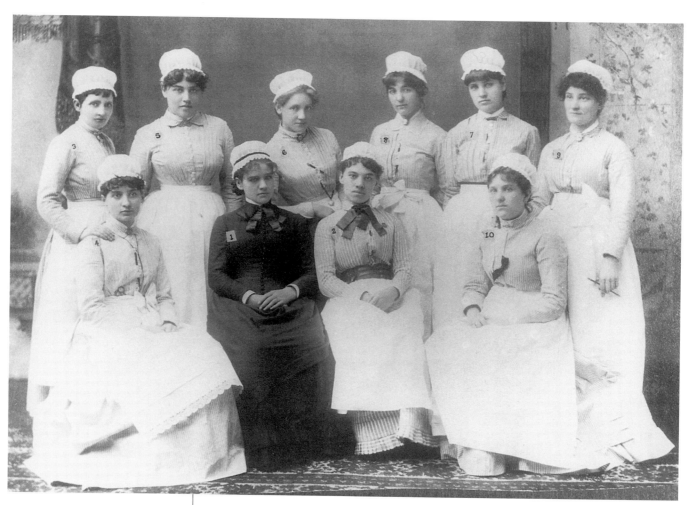

The first graduating class of nurses from City Hospital (Indianapolis) in 1885 (From the collection of the Wishard Nursing Museum)

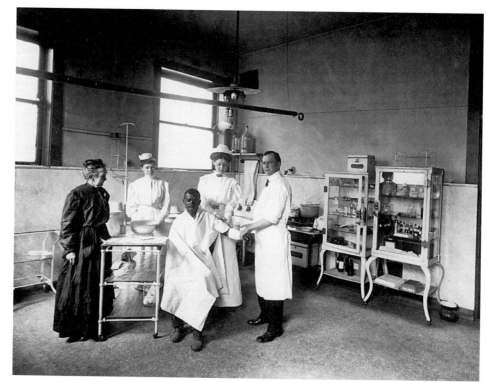

The City Hospital (Indianapolis) Dispensary in 1887. On the left in the dark uniform is Mrs. Peter Bryce, superintendent of nurses. She was often called Mother Bryce. Dr. Reid is dressing a patient's wound. Nurses were allowed to wear brooches and belt buckles, as noted on the nurse to Dr. Reid's right. (From the collection of the Wishard Nursing Museum)

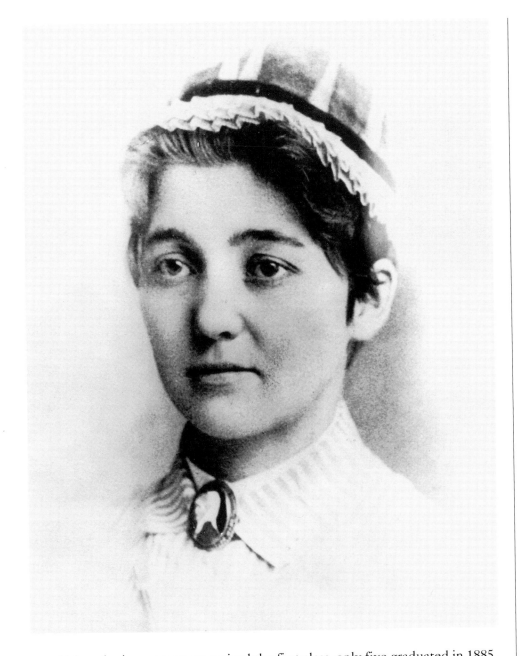

Margaret Iddings is recognized as Indiana's first professionally trained nurse. She graduated from City Hospital (Indianapolis) in 1885. (ISNA Archives)

Although nine women comprised the first class, only five graduated in 1885, following the two-year course of study. As in other schools, the nursing students were part of the hospital workforce and earned a small monthly payment for their services. They received eight dollars per month during the first year and twelve dollars per month during the second year, along with room and board in exchange for service. Faculty used an 1878 textbook titled the *Handbook of Nursing*, likely the manual that physicians and nurses from New Haven's Connecticut Training School wrote that year. Students also received lectures from the physicians on anatomy, physiology, and "materia medica" (pharmacology). Skills included cooking for the ill patient, giving baths and enemas, doing bandaging, applying dressings, making beds, providing a healthy environment, and making observations and reporting them to the doctor. Between 1885 and 1890, twenty-nine women graduated from the training school.[39]

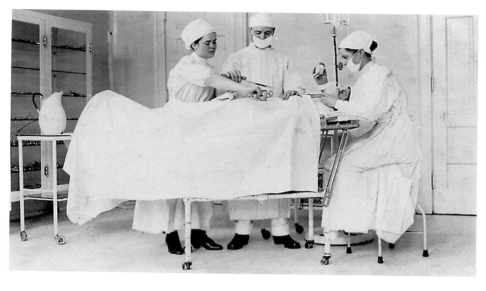

Nurses in the operating room, City Hospital (Indianapolis), in the early 1900s. The nurse at the head of the patient is anesthetizing with drop ether. (From the collection of the Wishard Nursing Museum)

Nursing reformers of the day believed that stipends furthered students' exploitation, and in 1889 Flower Mission administrators changed the students' pay to four dollars per month for the two years of study. This covered uniforms, books, and other personal expenses. The Annual Report noted that this "is in no wise intended as wages, it being considered that the education given is a full equivalent for their services." Typically students worked twelve-hour shifts (including nights after the first three months) with an hour off for dinner and additional time for exercise and rest. They had half a day off on Sunday, another half day during the week in the afternoon, and two weeks vacation each year. Upon graduation, nurses had a choice of working in hospitals, as district nurses, or as private-duty nurses in the home.[40]

As a benefit to its graduates, in 1890 the Flower Mission Training School opened a registry for private-duty nurses. In this way, the superintendent could keep lists of those nurses desiring private duty in order to help give them work. Registered nurses could receive $2.50 per day. Registries by other Indiana hospitals soon followed the same plan as the Flower Mission. In 1896 the Flower Mission Training School became a department of the Indianapolis City Hospital, necessitating a name change to Indianapolis City Hospital Training School for Nurses. This move also brought about an administrative change: the male superintendent of the hospital took charge of this department just as he did over all others in the hospital.[41] As the women at Flower Mission ceased their sponsorship, they did so at a time when male physicians and boards of trustees were increasingly gaining power in other hospitals.

By the end of 1899 several schools of nursing in Indiana had opened, i.e., Welborn Memorial Baptist Hospital School of Nursing in Evansville (1894), Protestant Deaconess Hospital School of Nursing in Evansville (1896), St. Vincent's Hospital School of Nursing in Indianapolis (1896), Memorial Hospital School of Nursing in South Bend (1896), Hope Hospital School of Nursing in Fort Wayne (1897), St. Elizabeth's Hospital Training School for Nurses in Lafayette (1897), Lafayette Home Hospital Training School for Nurses (1899), St. Stephen's (Reid Memorial) Hospital School of Nursing in Richmond (1899), and Union Hospital School of Nursing in Terre Haute (1900).[42] Students spent fifty to seventy hours a week in clinical training in addition to classes. Besides providing for hygiene and giving medications, they continued to do a great amount of housekeeping work. They also had office and switchboard duties, assisted in the pharmacy and laboratory, and did non-technical tasks in the X-ray department.[43]

The first national professional nursing organization was established in 1893 when nursing superintendents met at the Nursing Congress in Chicago during the World's Fair and Columbian Exposition. They formed the American Society of Superintendents of Training Schools for Nurses with the purpose of developing and maintaining a universal training standard. In 1897 individual nursing alumnae associations, aligned with hospitals and schools of nursing, joined to form the Nurses' Associated Alumnae of the United States and Canada. In Indiana, women formed an association for professional nurses known as "The Nightingales" in 1885. Four years later, trained nurses formed the Graduate Nurses Association in Indianapolis.[44]

In 1903 Civil War nurse Mary Livermore spoke at the Annual Convention of the Nurses' Associated Alumnae. She paid tribute to the new profession of nursing that had been sown from women's nursing experiences in the Civil War. By that time, American nursing had just witnessed what nurse historian Teresa E. Christy called the "Fateful Decade." The ten-year period between 1890 and 1900 saw the emergence of important nursing leaders, a proliferation of nurse training schools, and the establishment of local and national organizations.[45] Indiana remained right in the throes of it all.

————— • ————

Endnotes

[1] Elizabeth Moreland Wishard, *William Henry Wishard, A Doctor of the Old School* (Indianapolis: Hollenbeck Press, 1920), 278; Peggy B. Seigel, "She Went to War: Indiana Women Nurses in the Civil War," *Indiana Magazine of History* 86 (1990): 1–27; and Frank Moore, *Women of the War* (Hartford, CT: National Publishing Co. 1866), 333–340.

[2] Susan M. Reverby, *Ordered to Care—The Dilemma of American Nursing, 1850–1945* (Cambridge: Cambridge University Press, 1987), 11–16.

[3] Dorothy R. Russo, *One Hundred Years of Indiana Medicine, 1849–1949* (Indianapolis: Indiana State Medical Association), 4.

[4] Logan Esarey, *History of Indiana from its Exploration to 1922*, vol. 1 (Dayton, Ohio: Historical Publishing Co., 1922), 28; Barnhart and Riker, *Indiana to 1816*, 8.

[5] Hester Anne Hale, *Caring for the Community: The History of Wishard Hospital* (Indianapolis: Wishard Memorial Foundation, 1999), 10–12.

[6] Logan Esarey, *History of Indiana* (New York: Harcourt, Brace, 1922), 171.

[7] Hale, 12.

[8] George W. Adams, *Doctors in Blue: The Medical History of the Union Army in the Civil War* (Baton Rouge: Louisiana State University Press, 1952), 222.

[9] James M. McPherson, *Battle Cry of Freedom: The Civil War Era* (New York: Ballantine Books, 1988), 486.

[10] Philip A. Kalisch and Beatrice J. Kalisch, *The Advance of American Nursing* (Philadelphia: J. B. Lippincott Co., 1995), 38–53; and Barbra Mann Wall, "Grace under Pressure: The Nursing Sisters of the Holy Cross, 1861–1865," *Nursing History Review* 1 (1993): 72.

[11] Editorial, *Indianapolis Daily Journal*, 18 June 1861.

[12] Mother Mary Cecelia, diary, 15 May 1861, Archives of the Sisters of Providence of Saint-Mary-of-the-Woods, Indiana.

[13] Sister Eugenia Logan, *History of the Sisters of Providence of Saint-Mary-of-the-Woods*, vol. 2 (Terre Haute, IN: Moore-Langen Printing Co., 1978), 67.

[14] Editorial.

[15] *Indianapolis Daily Journal*, 23 March 1863.

[16] Ibid., 22 July 1864.

[17] Wall, 71–87.

[18] Olin D. Morrison, *Indiana's Care of Her Soldiers in the Field, 1861–1865* (Bloomington: Indiana University, 1926), 279.

[19] Adams, 7–8; and McPherson, 480–481.

[20] Seigel, 4–23; Morrison, 280; Wall, 73–74.

[21] Seigel, 11; Adams, 182; and Ann Douglas Wood, "The War within a War: Women Nurses in the Union Army," *Civil War History* 18 (1972): 197–212.

[22] Wall, 72.

[23] William Hannaman, *Indiana Sanitary Commission: Final Report of Officers, 1866* (Indiana State Archives, 18 August 1866).

[24] Reverby, 58.

[25] Dotaline Allen, *History of Nursing in Indiana* (Indianapolis: Wolfe Publishing, 1950), 7–13.

[26] Hale, 19.

[27] Betty Cotner Eller, and Virginia Maier Cafouros, ed., *110th Anniversary of the Wishard Memorial Hospital School of Nursing* (Indianapolis: private printing by authors, 1993), 2.

[28] Hale, 31.

[29] Ibid., 23.

[30] Allen, 13–22.

[31] *One Hundred Years Young—Anniversary Book 1878–1978* (Fort Wayne, Indiana: Parkview Hospital, 1978), Allen County Historical Society, Fort Wayne, Indiana.

[32] Allen, 13–22.

[33] Kalisch and Kalisch, 64–84; and Allen, 21.

[34]Reverby; and I. H. Robb, *Educational Standards for Nurses, With Other Addresses on Nursing Subjects* (New York: Garland Publishing Inc., 1985; original work published in 1907).

[35]E. F. Hodges's Letter to the Editor, *Indianapolis Journal*, Box 12, folder 9, Indiana Historical Society (hereafter cited as IHS).

[36]Allen, 34–35; *Annual Report: Flower Mission Training School for Nurses, January 1890* (Indianapolis: Reproduced by Marion County General Hospital, 1961), 20; and Hale.

[37]*Annual Report*, 12.

[38]Eller and Cafouros.

[39]Hale, 16–32; and *Annual Report Flower Mission*, 25.

[40]*Annual Report*, 14–17 (quotation on p. 16).

[41]Allen, 31–32; and Hale, 43–45.

[42]Allen, 51–53.

[43]Suzanne Parr and Toby Etchels, "Serving the Profession Since 1903: A Brief History of the Indiana State Nurses Association," *The Indiana Nurse* (1993): 63.

[44]Minutes of Graduate Nurses Association, Box 1, Folder 1, IHS.

[45]Teresa E. Christy, "Nurses in American History: The Fateful Decade, 1890–1900," *American Journal of Nursing* 75, No. 7 (1975): 1,163; and Kalisch and Kalisch, 55.

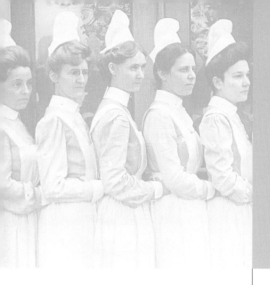

Chapter 2

"Forming a State Association in Indiana"
1900-1920

Barbra Mann Wall, Ph.D., R.N.

"In 1903, only one Alumnae in the State was affiliated with the National. To the Superintendent and this Alumnae the National appealed, asking them to do what they could toward forming a State Association in Indiana."[1] So wrote E. Gertrude Fournier, superintendent of Hope Hospital in Fort Wayne, Indiana, and a leader in the formation of the Indiana State Nurses Association (ISNA). Representing the state's first alumnae association from Hope Hospital, Fort Wayne, Mrs. Fournier was a delegate to the National Convention of the Nurses Associated Alumnae in 1903. Nursing leaders had called for the formation of state associations with the initial purpose of passing laws for the registration of nurses. At that time, many women were calling themselves "nurses." One leader wrote, "[T]he public are woefully ignorant in regard to the education and requirements of the modern trained nurse....But let any woman go into a community, adopt a nurse's uniform, and call herself a trained nurse, and her statement will be accepted without question by the majority of physicians and the public at large."[2] Indeed, no legal restrictions prevented any person from representing herself as a trained nursing graduate. State registration would establish fixed professional standards for nurses, impose order and uniformity to the profession, and protect the public.

Efforts to improve nursing at this time took place during the Progressive Era, a broad-based reform movement that spanned the 1890s and ended with America's entry into World War I. Influenced by the ills stemming from industrialization and urbanization, women spearheaded many projects, such as the settlement house movement, the National Consumer's League, and the Children's Bureau. Hundreds of hospitals grew under the sponsorship of religious orders, industrialists, women's organizations, ethnic groups, and committees of well-established elites.[3] The image of medicine improved with the establishment of the germ theory, scientific advances in diagnosis and treatment, and efficacy in the laboratory. Accompanying reform was a growing emphasis on professionalization with its imposition of standards and the licensing of personnel. In 1897 a law had established the Indiana State Board of Medical Registration and Examination.[4] The lack of uniform standards in nursing led to nursing leaders' efforts to do the same.

"Miss Johnson…Saved the Day": Early Organization of the ISNA

The basis of state organization in Indiana was the nurse training school alumnae associations. Encouraged by the national organization's charge, Mrs. Fournier and the Hope Hospital Alumnae Association issued circulars to as many hospitals as could be located where training schools existed, inviting nurses to attend a meeting at Hope Hospital on 3 September 1903. They also sent notices to the *American Journal of Nursing* (*AJN*), which had been established in 1900, and to major newspapers across the state. When the moment arrived, Mrs. Fournier addressed the meeting and presented the national association's request. The discussion did not go without difficulty; the motion to organize the state nurses association was "thoroughly discussed and finally carried." Elizabeth Johnson, a delegate from Indianapolis, played an important role. According to Dr. Maude McConnell, a medical doctor, nurse, and charter member of the ISNA, Mrs. Fournier often stated, "Miss Johnson…saved the day as they would not have had the courage to organize if no one had responded, so Indianapolis tipped the scales and made the ISNA materialize." Afterward, the women adopted a constitution and by-laws.[5]

On 27 November 1903 nurses from seven cities met to elect officers and form additional committees. The sixty-five attendees enrolled as charter members of the ISNA and elected E. Gertrude Fournier as the first president. Other officers included: M. Henderson of Union Hospital, Terre Haute, first vice president; Louise Hill, Fort Wayne, second vice president; Mary Scott, Indianapolis, secretary; and Florence Grant, City Hospital, Indianapolis, treasurer. Chairs of six standing committees—Nominations, Arrangements, Credentials, By-Laws, Legislation, and Publication—were appointed. After her installation, Mrs. Fournier addressed the group, "expressing her elation over the success of the organization and over the excellent prospects for the future."[6]

At the next meeting in February 1904, the association chose the motto, "Memor," Latin for "mindful." Nurses divided the state into thirteen districts for the purpose of caucusing and voted to have semiannual meetings at alternating

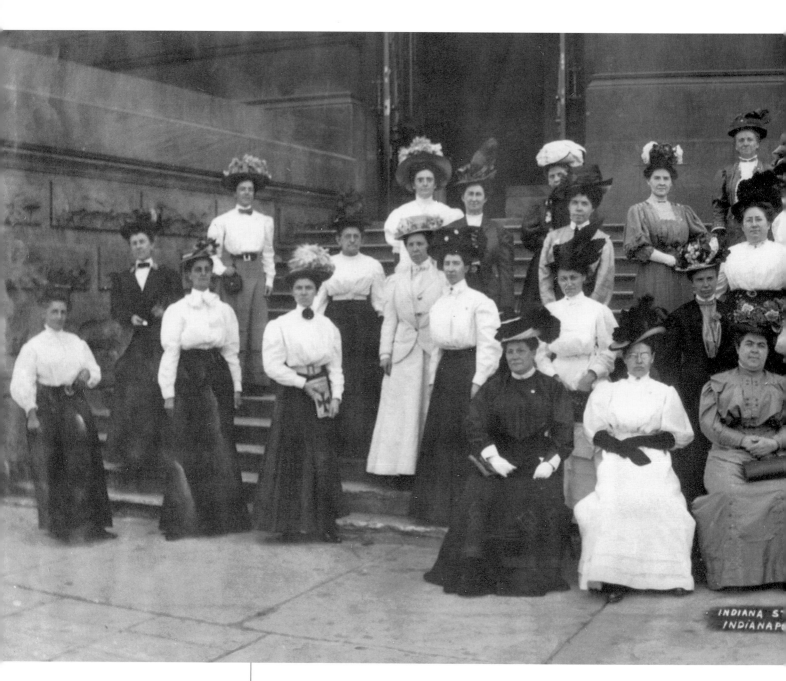

sites between the northern and southern parts of the state.[7] The local newspaper reported the following address by Mrs. Fournier: "The time has come when our profession will be recognized by law, and we should regulate these coming laws, rather than the physicians." She highlighted the nurse training school movement and noted, "The day of Sarah [Sairy] Gamp...passed a long time ago."[8] The ISNA incorporated on 4 March 1904 with the following purpose:

Indianapolis was the site for the 1908 ISNA Annual Meeting. While many of the members are not identified, the known delegates are: First row: 1. E. Gertrude Fournier, first president; 2. Anna Rein; 3. Mae Currie; 4. Edna Humphrey; 5. Mary Sollers; 6. Minnie Prange. Second row: 1. Frances Teague; 2. Frances Ott; 4. Florence Martin; 9. Stella Cotton; 14. May Rutan Baylor; 15. Mae Gentry. Third row: 2. Jeanette Miller; 7. Cora Nifer; 8. Elizabeth Johnson; 13. Cora Williams; 16. Miss Evans; 17. Ida McCaslin. (ISNA Archives)

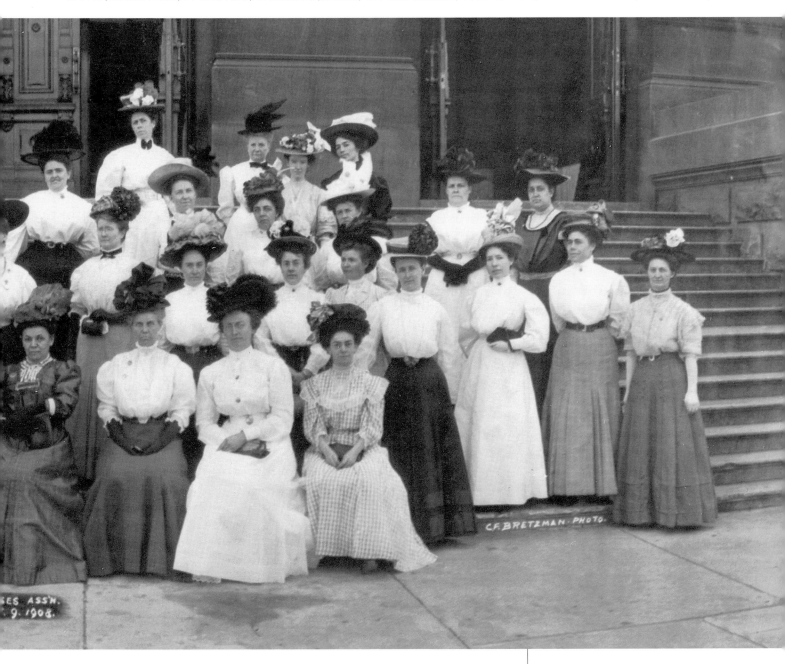

[T]he advancement of the educational and literary standard of nurses and nursing, the furtherance of the efficient and scientific care of the sick, to aid in the practice of medicine and surgery, the maintenance of the honor and character of the nursing profession and the furtherance of the cordial relations between the nurses of the State of Indiana and the nurses of other States and countries.[9]

This is the original incorporation certificate, issued in 1904 by the Indiana secretary of state, which established the Indiana State Nurses Association. The photo was enhanced to show the original text that was typed on the blank lines. The typewritten text has faded over the past one hundred years. (ISNA Archives)

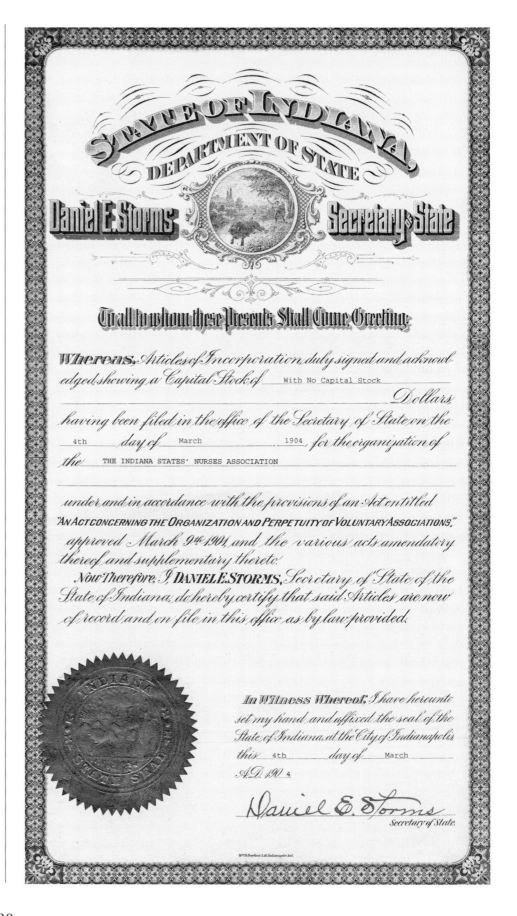

STATE OF INDIANA,

DEPARTMENT OF STATE

Daniel E. Storms

Secretary of State

To all to whom these Presents Shall Come, Greeting:

Whereas, Articles of Incorporation duly signed and acknowledged showing a Capital Stock of _With No Capital Stock_ Dollars, having been filed in the office of the Secretary of State on the _4th_ day of _March_ _1904_, for the organization of the _THE INDIANA STATES' NURSES ASSOCIATION_ under and in accordance with the provisions of an Act entitled "An Act concerning the Organization and Perpetuity of Voluntary Associations," approved March 9th 1901, and the various acts amendatory thereof and supplementary thereto:

Now Therefore, I, DANIEL E. STORMS, Secretary of State of the State of Indiana, do hereby certify that said Articles are now of record and on file in this office as by law provided.

In Witness Whereof, I have hereunto set my hand and affixed the seal of the State of Indiana, at the City of Indianapolis this _4th_ day of _March_ A.D. 190_4_.

Daniel E. Storms
Secretary of State.

28

The early alumnae associations joined as a body, but since there were only a few nurse training schools in Indiana at the time, most of the membership consisted of individual members. As training schools grew over the following decade, more alumnae associations were created. By 1907 the ISNA membership had risen to 146, and alumnae associations comprised much of the organization.[10] That year, they adopted a badge that distinguished them as members.

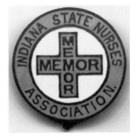

This was the original badge nurses received upon joining the Indiana State Nurses Association. (ISNA Archives)

To control the education of nurses, requirements for membership included graduation from acceptable nurse training schools. Members of the Indianapolis Graduate Nurses Association limited their group to Caucasians. In 1903 an African American nurse applied for membership. Minutes of the 7 October meeting noted, "[O]n account of the color line, the secretary was instructed to write to each nurse asking for her expression as to admitting her to membership." At the December meeting the voting revealed, "colored nurses debarred from membership in the association."[11]

After 1890 segregation had spread under the rubric of the slogan, "separate but equal." In many parts of the country, particularly in the South, it extended to facilities such as restaurants and public transportation. It culminated in 1896 with the Supreme Court decision in the case *Plessy v. Ferguson*, which upheld the legality of segregation as long as the facilities themselves were equal. Segregation also applied to many professional organizations. Although black nurses supported the adoption of legislation to enhance nursing standards, many were unable to secure membership in their state associations, and as a result, could not join the American Nurses Association (ANA). In 1908 they formed their own professional organization, the National Association of Colored Graduate Nurses. Darlene Clark Hine argues that some ANA leaders

A 1904 receipt from the Indiana Secretary of State acknowledging the incorporation of the Indiana State Nurses Association. The filing fee was $6.50. Note the receipt was printed in the 1890s and that date was corrected to reflect the 1904 filing date. (ISNA files)

saw the need to integrate black nurses into the ANA, but "their less progressive and more economically vulnerable membership thought otherwise." Had leaders actively pursued integration, they would have alienated most of the members, which they were not willing to do. Thus, future recruitment and growth of the professional organizations "dictated a careful adherence to the color line."[12] No information is available in the ISNA records as to the association's policy.

"If I Was Acquainted with Any Person of Influence": Nurse Registration Legislation

For the state association, the most important business transacted over the first year was to secure a nursing registration bill. In 1903 North Carolina was the first state to pass a registration law, followed by New York, New Jersey, Virginia, and Maryland. Indiana became the sixth state when it passed its law in 1905, and it was the first Midwestern state to enact such a law.[13] Sarah Belk Brown, chair of the Legislative Committee, and five other members drafted the bill to which Dr. William Niles Wishard made significant revisions. From the beginning, the ISNA sought support from influential persons and organizations. Mrs. Brown highlighted the Legislative Committee's work in the following report:

> The probabilities are that some may wish to know of the preliminary work done in getting the Bill ready for presentation; of course there must be a certain amount of support from the physicians and surgeons. We called personally on a number of these and the measure met with their approval and their support was cheerfully given….Some physicians do not approve of any medical legislation, hence didn't see the need of legislation for nurses. I know that quite a few of the physicians did very efficient work for us among the members of the General Assembly. Some deserving especial mention are Dr. W. N. Wishard; he being well known in medical legislation was able to influence many people; Drs. S. N. Cunningham, J. H. Oliver, Ross Robertson, E. F. Hodges; Dr. Wishard having a way of reaching so many as he was urging the law needed to be changed.[14]

Members of the ISNA aggressively sought this support. In late 1904 Dr. Maude McConnell presented the proposed bill to the Indianapolis Medical Society. The physicians passed resolutions endorsing the bill, and two Indiana medical journals published supporting editorials. On 19 December 1904 Sarah

Brown, Gertrude Fournier, and ISNA secretary Miss F. M. Grant mailed a copy of the bill to all nurses whose addresses were known. They also sent a circular letter laying out the object of state registration.

Sarah Brown reported that, at the same time, the ISNA leaders mailed "to each senator and representative at his home address, a copy of the Bill and with this we enclosed a list of the names of the physicians who had given their support and a circular letter asking their favorable consideration….In any case if I was acquainted with any person of influence or knew anybody who might know someone who could bring any influence upon legislators, their interests were promptly enlisted."[15]

On 11 January 1905 State Representative William Bosson introduced the bill to the Indiana General Assembly. The bill required the registration of all trained nurses; provided for a Board of Examiners, with the ISNA nominating twelve and the governor appointing five members; fixed the number and qualifications of the Board; and provided for the registering of nurses with penalties for any violations of the act. The bill was referred to the House Committee on Medical Health and Vital Statistics and became known as House Bill 15. A group of the ISNA nurses lobbied with this committee to emphasize the importance of such a measure.[16] When the governor conferred with the committee, however, he objected to the ISNA making

Circular letter to Indiana nurses in support of the registration bill, 1905

1905

In the Interest of the Bill for State Registration to be Introduced at the Present Session of the Legislature by

The Indiana State Nurses' Association

TO THE NURSES OF THE STATE OF INDIANA:

Nursing is a profession requiring a high degree of ability and training; in view of the responsibility of the duties of the graduate nurse, it would appear to be as essential on general principles that the qualifications of the nurse should be determined and fixed by registration as the qualifications of the physician, pharmacist or dentist should be fixed by law.

It would also appear that the minimum qualification of the nurse should be ascertained by a Board of Examiners chosen from the Nursing profession, thus following the precept given by older professions of Medicine, Pharmacy and Dentistry.

For this object a bill has been prepared to establish a uniform standard of education, fitness and ability. The substance of this bill, briefly stated is as follows:

Prior to January 1st, 1906, all nurses of good standing who possess the following qualifications, may register without examination.

Graduates from all general hospitals giving a two years course; all nurses who are in training in a general hospital at time of passage of this act.

Graduates of special hospitals, who have been nursing five years; or who shall obtain six months additional training in an approved general hospital.

After June 1st, 1908, a state examination will be required. The applicant must be twenty-three years old, of good moral character and possess the equivalent of a high-school education, and be a graduate from a training-school connected with a general hospital of good standing, where three years of training and systematic instruction are given in the hospital.

The passage of this bill shall not affect or apply to the gratuitous nursing of the sick by friends or members of the family or any persons nursing the sick for hire, who do not assume to be trained or registered nurses.

It will give a legal status so that the professional nurse will be the registered nurse. It will prevent a probationer who was not accepted because of unfitness, or a pupil who was dismissed for just cause, from posing as a graduate nurse. It will prevent the unqualified and unscrupulous from palming themselves upon the public as duly qualified graduate nurses.

Important information concerning the need of registration may be found on pages 771 to 785 in the Convention number (July 1904) of The American Journal of Nursing.

Forward any ideas that may strengthen this movement to the Legislative Committee of the Indiana State Nurses' Association, and remember the words of our great leader Florence Nightingale:

"Nursing is an art; and if it is to be made an art requires as exclusive a devotion, as hard a preparation, as any painter's or sculptor's work, for what is having to do with dead canvas or cold marble compared with having to do with the living body, the temple of God's Spirit."

PRESIDENT—MRS. E. G. FOURNIER,
Hope Hospital, Fort Wayne, Ind.

SECRETARY—MISS F. M. GRANT,
City Hospital, Indianapolis, Ind.

CHAIRMAN OF LEGISLATIVE COMMITTEE—MRS. CHARLES A. BROWN,
3010 N. Capitol Ave., Indianapolis, Ind.

twelve nominations from which he appointed a board of five. Hence, the committee struck the clause and gave greater appointive power to the governor.

More opposition arose in the Senate. One senator argued that the bill was discriminatory in its favor of graduates of established training schools connected with general hospitals. It would "bar nurses who, although able to practice their profession intelligently, might not be able to pass a technical examination required under the provisions of the bill." He recommended that any nurse of seven years' experience, with three spent in general or special hospitals, be eligible for registration. Another amendment reduced the length of nurses' training required for application, after 1 June 1908, to two years rather than three, which the ISNA wanted. Some senators argued that these amendments would lower standards, and Bosson and three physicians made speeches for the bill. Nevertheless, the amendments were adopted. Nurses continued their aggressive lobbying; indeed, some legislators criticized their presence at almost every session of the Senate. Sarah Brown commented that discussion over the bill "was quite warm and to the nurses present quite exciting."[17]

At the same time, other nurses resisted the bill's passage. One objected to the Board of Examiners consisting of women. "You cannot tell when a woman will get foolish nor how foolish she will get." She preferred working under the State Medical Board.[18] The *AJN* reported that "bitter opposition" arose in Indiana from special schools and untrained women.[19] Indeed, internal conflicts within nursing accompanied the movement for registration. As new standards restricted access to the nursing profession, some nurses already working were left out.

Opposition in Indiana proved to be minimal, however, and House Bill 15 governing the registration of nurses passed in the Senate 38–3 and 79–10 in the House. Governor Frank Hanley signed it on 27 February 1905. It created the State Board of Examination and Registration for Nurses, to which the governor appointed four nurses and one female physician. It also provided a period during which nurses with varying lengths of training could be registered without examination, thereby protecting suitable nurses who trained or practiced prior to the legal enactment.[20] Sarah Brown and other ISNA leaders considered the lowering of educational standards as a "molestation" of the bill. Mrs. Brown later admitted, "But even these concessions were less than was expected we might have to make." Upon reflection of the process, she stated, "I think we experienced less attack upon measure in the House as we had personal friends there who could be constantly on the outlook for our interests."[21] Indeed, networking with those in power proved extremely beneficial. In 1921 an amendment to the law gave the ISNA the right to submit a list of names to the governor from which he selected names for the State Board.

In January 1906 the *AJN* reported 275 nurses had received certificates of registration in Indiana, although the numbers were fewer than in some other states. By the next year, more than 600 Indiana nurses had obtained registration.[22] After 1 June 1908 the law required State Board examinations. Until that time, nurses merely had to meet age and training or experience requirements to be registered. The Nurse Practice Act has been amended a number of times, and the ISNA has successfully defended it against other amendments.

Leaders in the ISNA and other state and national associations accurately identified some of the nursing profession's problems: the exploitative apprenticeship system of training and the vulnerability of patients to incompetent care from poorly trained nurses. In addition to increasing nursing standards, association leaders' strong contribution was in their extension of professional advantages, previously claimed by white male elites, to women. Their solutions, however, also created some problems for those left out, and these women often sought other means of legitimacy.[23] In 1910 a few nurses from a leading Indiana city joined a trades union. Correspondence between Indiana nursing leaders and Lavinia Dock, an early nurse feminist who was instrumental in establishing the national nurses' association, revealed the following response from Dock. She cautioned them to avoid assuming "an exclusive attitude....I myself feel that trades unions are just as worthy of respect and recognition as any other associations in the world....But I would point out that these women are driven to ally themselves with the trades union because they have not had the education that would enable them to join the registered nurses," mainly because they had received their education from correspondence schools. She predicted, however, that if doctors "keep on showing an absolute lack of ethics and loyalty to nurses that all nurses will finally join trades unions in order to strengthen their economic position."[24]

Efforts to upgrade the nursing profession also included measures to improve its nurses. Leaders consistently called for more "cultured women" to fill its ranks. In 1907 one nurse noted that educational standards and other requirements were needed not only to protect the public but also to get the highest class of applicants possible. "It was in order to put the nurse on a higher plane that we urged the enactment of the law requiring all trained nurses to register."[25]

The professionalization of nursing offered many aspiring women opportunities for occupational mobility, and it raised the overall status of nursing. At the same time, the professional association engendered friendships among women and furnished them opportunities to develop new skills.[26] Nurses often described their qualifications in distinctly feminine tones. Allie Butler, in a paper presented at an ISNA meeting, indicated that in their public presentation of themselves, nurses should have a quiet touch, pure character, pleasing manners, ready sympathy, and a polite, agreeable, and kind personality. Yet, refusing to be limited by gender conventions, she added, "It has sometimes been claimed that all women make good nurses by virtue of their womanhood, but this is not true....Nursing is a profession requiring a high degree of ability and training."[27] Indeed, good intentions did not compensate for a lack of intelligence or skill.

Educational Standards

Shortly after the passage of the Nurse Practice Act in 1905, problems became apparent for the Indiana State Board of Examination and Registration. Varied curriculums and lengths of nurses' training made it difficult for the Board to decide who was eligible for registration. Since Indiana membership in the American Society of Superintendents of Training Schools for Nurses was limited, the elevation of standards for education fell to the ISNA and the State Board. In 1907, the State Board set up a uniform curriculum.

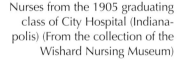

Nurses from the 1905 graduating class of City Hospital (Indianapolis) (From the collection of the Wishard Nursing Museum)

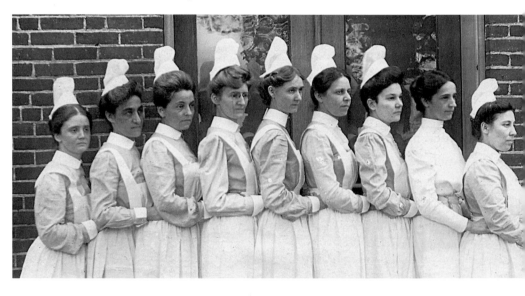

State Board member Lizzie Cox undertook an inspection of hospitals and training schools in the state in 1908.[28] She reported her findings to the ISNA Annual Convention in Indianapolis that year. Whereas in 1905 there were fewer than twenty nurse training schools in Indiana, by 1908, thirty-eight out of seventy hospitals and sanitariums inspected conducted their own schools.[29] Some of these included St. Joseph's Hospital School of Nursing, South Bend (1907), and Methodist Hospital School of Nursing, Indianapolis (1908). Hope Hospital in Fort Wayne was the only one with eight-hour workdays and three shifts. The largest hospital and training school was the 180-bed City Hospital

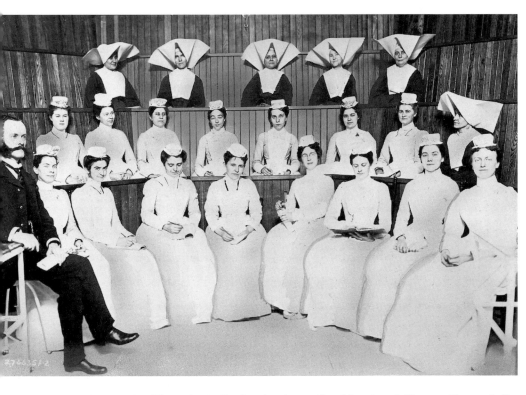

St. Vincent's Hospital (Indianapolis) nurses in 1902 (ISNA Collection M0380, Indiana Historical Society)

of Indianapolis. Two Catholic institutions, St. Mary's of Evansville and St. Vincent's in Indianapolis, were next in size. As a result of the inspection, Miss Cox recommended more classroom instruction, especially in dietetics. She insisted on "class work and lectures; we want not better trained nurses but more practical nurses having a more thorough knowledge of the textbooks." She also maintained that each nurse training school should have a graduate at its head, and that no hospital should have a training school unless it supported ten beds.[30] Miss Cox did another survey in 1910 to determine if schools were concurring with the standard curriculum. Courses were gradually brought into compliance, solving some of the problems associated with registration.[31]

In 1909 the Indiana State Society of Superintendents of Training Schools was formed. When the American Society of Superintendents changed its name in 1912 to the National League for Nursing Education, the Indiana organization followed suit and became the Indiana State League for Nursing Education.[32]

In 1912 nursing leader Mary Adelaide Nutting's report to the United States Bureau of Education noted more than 1,100 nursing schools in the United States. Describing Indiana programs for the year 1910–1911, she documented twenty-eight schools in hospitals that had bed capacities of ten or more (excluding schools connected with hospitals for mental disorders). In these, 488 students were enrolled, and 135 had graduated during the year. Requirements for admission were anywhere from eighth grade or common school education, to high school, reflecting Indiana's registration law that specified the educational requirement to be "high school or its equivalent." By comparison, of the thirty-one states with registration laws, eighteen had no educational requirement at all. Nine of the twenty-eight schools had only two years of training, while for the majority, the academic term was three years. In 1913 the Indiana Nurse Practice Act was amended to require a three-year course of instruction.

According to Nutting's study, Indiana nursing students compared favorably in other areas. Ages ranged from nineteen to thirty-five, typical of other states. Indianapolis City Hospital and St. Vincent's Hospital enrolled and graduated the most students. Only seven schools reported requiring eight hours of duty, while twelve had nine hours and the remainder, ten to twelve hours. These findings were somewhat better than schools in other states, where nearly half required students to be on duty ten hours or more daily, irrespective of classroom lectures or study. Nutting considered the long hours of work an "intolerable offense against the principles for which the hospital and training school are standing in modern society."[33] While laws raised standards of training and established uniform requirements for nursing registration, improvement clearly was still needed.

African American women had few opportunities to study nursing. In Indianapolis, racism prevented blacks from gaining access to city hospitals, and African American women's clubs spent great efforts toward establishing separate institutions. Women from various organizations created a tuberculosis sanitarium and other hospitals and provided funds for African American women to obtain nurses' training. These hospitals were short-lived, however, due to inadequate facilities and lack of funding.[34]

"Not Gun Powder but Education and Right Living": The ISNA and Political Activism

The ISNA soon took on pressure group tactics. In 1909 a representative from the Women's Christian Temperance Union asked for the nurses' help to "down the liquor traffic and its attending evils," and members endorsed a resolution in 1909. In 1910 after a request for help from the Indiana State Medical Association, the ISNA members urged the Indiana General Assembly to enact a law requiring medical inspection of school children to prevent blindness stemming from neonatal defects. The ISNA members sent copies of the resolution to the governor, secretary of state, lieutenant governor, and each member of the general assembly then in session. They urged their own ISNA members and their affiliates to write their representatives and were rewarded when the bill passed that same year.[35]

Public health nursing was a frequent topic discussed at meetings. It was the elite area in which nurses could work. In 1908 members formed a Public Health Committee within the ISNA and worked toward the prevention of tuberculosis (TB). Throughout the following decade, they presented papers at meetings, invited the president of the state Anti-Tuberculosis Association to speak, endorsed the movement to erect a state TB hospital, participated in education projects, and backed the formation of a state public health association. In their campaign to eradicate disease from overcrowded living conditions, these public-spirited nurses supported district nurses in caring for the impoverished sick at home. This involved education in good health habits and proper hygiene, as long as it was undertaken with some degree of sensitivity to the tenants. A presenter at a 1912 ISNA meeting advocated that visiting nurses "must get acquainted with tenants before much can be accomplished."[36] At the same meeting, Dr. Maude McConnell gave a paper on TB. Placing the dangers of the disease into perspective, she referred to the tragic sinking of the luxury ship *Titanic* just one week before when more than 1,500 people died. "The loss of life on the *Titanic*," she stated, "was not so great as the loss of life from disease; our weapons for fighting are not gun powder but education and right living."[37]

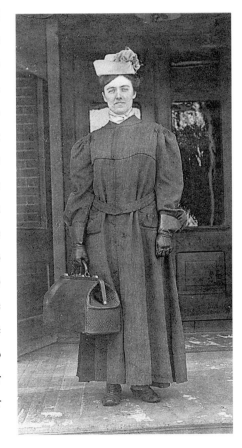

Mabel Goodale, a public health nurse from Indianapolis, in the 1920s (From the collection of the Wishard Nursing Museum)

As messengers of cleanliness and character, nurses proved central to the modern public health campaign. In 1912 they formed the National Organization for Public Health Nursing. In 1916 Public Health became a separate section in the ISNA. Speeches at the ISNA meetings were explicit in expressing concerns about disease and called on nurses to assume greater responsibility in this arena.

The ISNA demonstrated a wide range of interests in the Progressive Era's reform movements and allied with individual reformers and women's organizations such as the elite Woman's Department Club in Indianapolis. In 1905 Indiana reformer May Wright Sewall, an invited speaker at the ISNA Annual Meeting, called on nurses to "ameliorate the conditions of the civilization that cultivates the offenses of disease."[38] Carolyn Barlett Crane from Kalamazoo, Michigan, was a leader in civic improvements and a national consultant on sanitary reform. As a guest speaker at the 1907 convention, she emphasized the role of the trained nurse in almshouse reform, and she convinced members to appoint a committee to meet with the Women's Federation of Clubs to address the matter. The Women's Federation of Clubs, of which the ISNA was an affiliate member, joined women's clubs all over Indiana under one forum. These women persevered to create social change before they attained suffrage and access to party politics.[39]

As it was, the ISNA had begun discussing the woman suffrage issue at its 1911 Annual Convention. The association invited Sophia Palmer, first editor of the *AJN*, to speak on the topic. She related that she had been opposed to woman suffrage until she became a member of New York's Board of Nurse Examiners and tried to get legislation passed that benefited the nursing profession. "A man with a vote," she stated, "had more influence with legislators than a whole crowd of women without votes."[40] Indeed, as nurses learned how important suffrage would be to their profession, many engaged in activities to bring it to fruition. In 1912 Grace Julian Clarke, a leading social reformer and women's activist, addressed the ISNA Annual Convention. While woman suffrage "would not bring about the millennium," it would enable "better educational interests and better social conditions....It is not a question about warfare between men and women. It is civilization against barbarism, and progress against stagnation." Drawing upon historical assumptions associating women with the domestic "sphere," at least in white middle-class homes, Clarke continued, "Women can no longer protect the sanctity of their home unless they have a vote in the making of the laws of our country."[41]

At the 1912 semiannual meeting in April, the ISNA endorsed suffrage: "If the subject of woman's suffrage came up [at the national meeting], it was moved and carried that our State Association stands for suffrage."[42] The Nurses Associated Alumnae, reorganized in 1911 to become the American Nurses Association (ANA), endorsed a woman suffrage resolution at its 1912 Annual Convention. The ANA then represented American nurses at the International Council of Nurses meeting in Cologne, Germany, that year and supported an international woman suffrage resolution.[43]

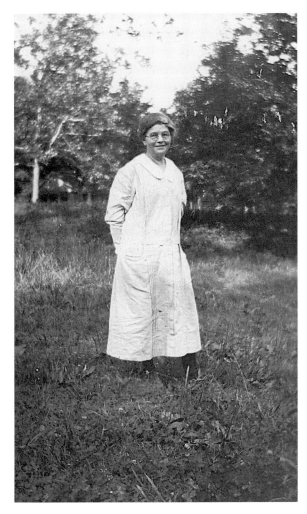

Anna Rein in 1928. A graduate of City Hospital (Indianapolis) in 1899, she held numerous offices in the ISNA, including president from 1912–1914. (ISNA Collection M0380, Indiana Historical Society)

The ISNA nurses made special efforts to set standards for themselves. In 1914 they developed a Code of Ethics detailing articles on loyalty, engagements, and the duties of the nurse to patients, the hospital, the public, and to physicians.[44] Red Cross work was another topic of interest, and members formed a committee to recruit for Red Cross nursing. In 1912 the ISNA invited Jane Delano, chair of the Red Cross Nursing Service, to speak at its annual meeting. Appeals for the Red Cross Nurse Corps continued until after World War I. Other subjects addressed at meetings were private-duty nursing, problems with registries, and later, questions over the twelve-hour day instead of the usual twenty hours. In 1914 the association asked Mrs. Albion Fellows Bacon, who had led a campaign for housing and tenement reform, to address members at the semi-annual meeting. Her topic, "The Relation of Health to the Home," emphasized the positive influence of home nursing. The nurse was an educator, a member of the board of health, and a "life preserver." Thus, through its organization and alliances with other women, the ISNA was able to participate in the women's movement and the reform community for the betterment of nurses, their profession, and their patients.

ISNA members enjoy the 1915 biennial convention in Terre Haute. (ISNA Collection M0380, Indiana Historical Society)

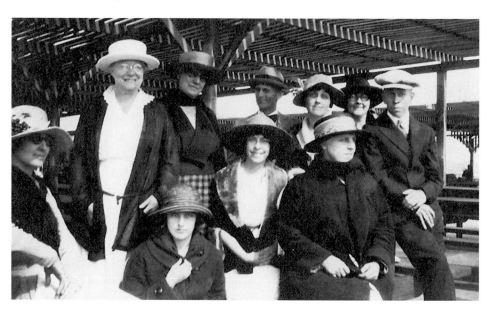

"Spread upon the Records": The ISNA during World War I

Serving under the Red Cross banner, nurses from Indiana cared for the casualties of World War I. The Red Cross had been the unofficial reserve of the Army Nurse Corps, and when the European war began in 1914 and more nurses were needed, the Red Cross furnished them. Four Indiana nurses went to Austria in 1915. On 6 April 1917 President Woodrow Wilson signed the declaration of war, and the United States began a huge campaign to support the Allied cause. Among others, ISNA members June Gray, Katherine Kreutzer, Alma Scott, and Aline Mergy served in base hospitals in France between 1917 and 1919, while Anna Rein was a Red Cross supervisor in Mississippi.[45]

The ISNA joined in the wartime effort at home by donating money to the Red Cross. Members also cooperated with the National Council of Defense to complete a census of nurses in the state. At the 1917 Annual Convention, a guest speaker talked on "topics nearest our hearts...the beauty of service at home and abroad." Nurses sang patriotic songs, purchased a liberty bond through a local woman's club, and voted to send Christmas cards to nurses abroad. An unidentified individual sang, "Keep the Home Fires Burning." It was announced that six more nurses were preparing for Red Cross duty. At the semiannual meeting in April 1918, Carolyn Schoemaker, a dean at Purdue University, urged the nurses to buy more liberty bonds, use thrift stamps, and practice economy in their clothing. A leading Red Cross representative from Indiana spoke of the great need for more nurses. She ardently claimed, "It is a magnificent privilege to be an American nurse at this time."[46]

At the war's end, the chair of the Indiana State Council of National Defense addressed the ISNA Annual Convention on problems that the conflict had brought. Tuberculosis cases were increasing. There had been 4,000 deaths from TB in 1918 alone, and 400 soldiers were discharged from the Army due to the disease. In addition, many men returned from the war needing psychiatric help. The Red Cross Committee's report was also revealing: nearly 500 nurses from Indiana had signed up, with many being in foreign service. The disastrous influenza epidemic of 1918 and 1919 had especially tested the nation's health, and the Public Health Committee reported that county emergency hospitals had been established.

Sadly, twelve nurses from Indiana died in service to their country, either in the military zone, army camps, or during the influenza epidemic. In their honor, members of the ISNA listed their names and adopted the following resolution:

> *Whereas, the loss of their unequalled services and valuable example will be deeply felt by the nursing profession,*
>
> *Be it resolved that we, the members of the Indiana State Nurses Association, regret their untimely deaths and extend to their families our sincere condolences and Be it resolved that copies of this resolution be sent to their families and that it be spread upon the records of this association.*[47]

Changes in Organization

Throughout the war and afterward, the ISNA continued its association with influential women's clubs. It was particularly active in public health work, with clubwomen helping to place nurses in needed public health areas. The highly visible work of new female wageworkers, clubwomen, and women mobilized into wartime service finally helped to secure the Nineteenth Amendment to the Constitution in 1920 that legalized women's right to vote.[48]

During the war years, nursing school enrollments increased across the country. Several of these were Catholic institutions under the direction of nuns. To keep pace with the hospital and nursing reform movement, sisters, priests, and physicians had formed a separate professional organization, the Catholic Hospital Association (CHA), in 1915. Although priests held the highest leadership positions until the 1960s, sisters served on the CHA executive board, headed committees, participated in conventions, and set standards for Catholic nursing education.[49] While religious rules forbade some sisters from serving in secular organizations, other nuns were not so restricted and they were both members and officers in the ISNA.

The Indiana State Conference of the Catholic Hospital Association held its annual meeting in 1922 at St. Elizabeth's Hospital in Lafayette. (Photo courtesy of Sisters of St. Francis of Perpetual Adoration, Mishawaka)

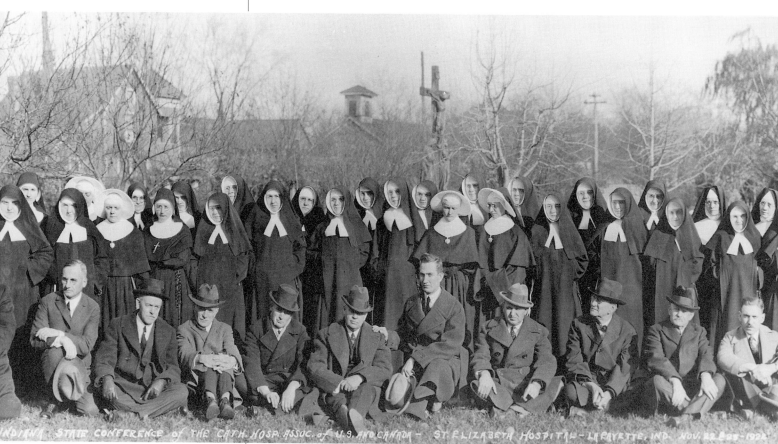

In 1918 the ANA revised its bylaws, making the state association the sole unit of membership. As a result, state associations reorganized and adopted a district plan of representation, and Indiana created four districts. Each district elected officers, wrote constitutions and bylaws, held regular meetings, and carried out the work of the state association at the local level. Representatives of the districts went as delegates to the annual meetings of the state and national associations. Bylaws of the ANA also specified that a nurse first had to join her alumnae association and then automatically became a member of the district. Dues included representation in the district, state, and national associations and were $4.50 in 1919.[50]

The ISNA continued its collaborative work with other organizations. In 1919 it supported the National League for Nursing Education's campaign for shorter working hours. It held affiliations with nine different organizations, including the International Council of Nurses, the National Council of Women, the Women's Joint Congressional Committee, and the General Federation of Women's Clubs. The ISNA grew from 65 charter members in 1903 to 1,120 members in 1925. By then it was an integral part of the ANA.

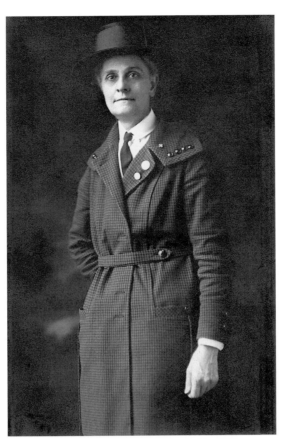

Frances M. Ott (1864-1954) was an active member of ISNA for many years. She was a champion of private duty nurses and was called the "Florence Nightingale of Private Duty." Her many nursing experiences also included "quarantine nursing" and Red Cross Nurse Corps during World War I. In May 1980, the Wishard Memorial School of Nursing Educational Building was renamed Frances M. Ott Building. ISNA started the Frances M. Ott Membership Award in 1955. It was given to the district achieving the highest potential of its membership. Source: Wishard Nursing Museum (ISNA Collection M0380, Indiana Historical Society)

Endnotes

[1] E. Gertrude Fournier, "How We Laid the Foundation of Our State Nurses Society in Indiana," written for the Twenty-Third Annual Convention of the ISNA, Box 12, folder 9, IHS.

[2] "The Editor," *AJN* 1, no. 2 (November 1900):166.

[3] Rosemary Stevens, *In Sickness and in Wealth: American Hospitals in the Twentieth Century* (Baltimore and London: Johns Hopkins University Press, 1989; repr. 1999), 17, 105.

[4] Clifton J. Phillips, *Indiana in Transition: The Emergence of an Industrial Commonwealth, 1880–1920* (Indianapolis: Indiana Historical Bureau and Indiana Historical Society, 1968), 473.

[5] Fournier; and Maude W. McConnell to Miss June Gray, 20 April (no year), Box 12, folder 9, IHS.

[6] 1903 ISNA Minutes, Box 2, folder 1, IHS. Quotation is in "Official Reports of Societies— Fort Wayne, Ind.," *AJN* 4, no. 4 (January 1904): 314.

[7] 1904 ISNA Minutes, IHS.

[8] Typed copy of newspaper article, "Indiana Nurses Will Demand Registration," sometime around February 22, 1904, Box 12, folder 9, IHS.

[9] Article I, "Articles of Incorporation," Box 10, folder 10, IHS.

[10] Mary M. Schroder, "History of the Indiana State Nurses' Association" (Master of Arts Thesis, University of Chicago, 1958), p. 6; and "Official Reports," *AJN* 7, no. 11 (August 1907): 808.

[11] Minutes of the Indianapolis Graduate Nurses Association, 7 October 1903, and 10 December 1903, Box 1, folder 1, IHS.

[12] Darlene Clark Hine, *Black Women in White: Racial Conflict and Cooperation in the Nursing Profession, 1890–1950* (Bloomington and Indianapolis: Indiana University Press, 1989), 115.

[13] Louie Croft Boyd, *State Registration for Nurses* (Philadelphia: W. B. Saunders Company, 1915); Sophia F. Palmer, "The Effect of State Registration Upon Training Schools," *AJN* 5 (1905): 657; and Maude W. McConnell, typed copy of report, Box 12, folder 9, IHS.

[14] Sarah Brown, "Report of the Chairman of the Legislative Committee," April 1905, IHS.

[15] Ibid.

[16] Ibid., and 1904 ISNA Minutes, Box 2, folder 1, IHS.

[17] Copy of "Trained Nurse Bill Has Narrow Escape," and typed copy of "For Registration of Nurses" in Box 12, folder 9, IHS.

[18] Typed copy of "Woman Wants Male Board," Box 12, folder 9, IHS.

[19] "Progress of State Registration," *AJN* 5, no. 7 (April, 1905): 414.

[20] "Official Reports, The Indiana Bill for the State Registration of Nurses," *AJN* 5, no. 7 (April 1905): 465–66; and 1905 ISNA Minutes (Semi-Annual Meeting), Box, 2, folder 1, IHS.

[21] Brown.

[22] "Progress of State Registration," *AJN* 6, no. 4 (January 1906): 213; and "Official Reports," *AJN* 7, no. 11 (August 1907): 808.

[23] Barbara Melosh, *"The Physician's Hand": Work Culture and Conflict in American Nursing* (Philadelphia: Temple University Press, 1982), 22, 34.

[24] Lavinia Dock to Miss Currie, 13 June 1910, Box 11, folder 10, IHS. See also "A Union in Indiana, Nurses Affiliated with the A.F. of L. Still Speak of Their 'Practice,'" copy of newspaper article, 1910, Box 11, folder 10, IHS.

[25] 1907 ISNA Minutes; "Ft. Wayne Chosen as Next Meeting Place," n.d., Box 2, folder 1, IHS.

[26] Julia Kirk Blackwelder, *Now Hiring: The Feminization of Work in the United States, 1900–1995* (College Station: Texas A&M University Press, 1997).

[27] Allie Butler, paper presented at 1907 (Semi-Annual) ISNA Meeting, Box 2, folder 1, IHS.

[28] 1908 ISNA Minutes, Box 2, folder 1, IHS; and Schroder, 14–17.

[29] Brown; Lizzie M. Cox, "Inspector's Report of Hospital Training Schools," 12 September 1908, Box 12, folder 9, IHS.

[30] Ibid.

[31] 1919 ISNA Minutes, Box 2, folder 3; typed history of the ISNA, Box 12, folder 9, IHS; and Schroder, 16–17.

[32] Dotaline E. Allen, "History of Nursing in Indiana," in D. Russo, ed., *One Hundred Years of Indiana Medicine, 1849–1949* (Indianapolis: Indiana State Medical Association, 1950), 137.

[33] M. Adelaide Nutting, *Educational Status of Nursing, Bulletin #7* (Washington, DC: Government Printing Office, 1912), 7–97. Quotation is on p. 33. Indiana statistics are on pp. 67–68.

[34] Anita Ashendel, "'Women as Force' in Indiana History," in *The State of Indiana History, 2000*, ed. Robert M. Taylor (Indianapolis: Indiana Historical Society, 2001), 23.

[35] 1908–1910 ISNA Minutes, IHS.

[36] Excerpts from paper, "Visiting Nurse and the Boarding House," noted in 1912 ISNA Minutes (Semi-Annual Meeting), Box 2, folder 1, IHS.

[37] Ibid.

[38]1905 ISNA Minutes, Box 2, folder 1, IHS.

[39]Ashendel, 16–17.

[40]Sophia Palmer, "A Retrospect and a Forecast," presented at the Ninth Annual Convention of the ISNA, noted in 1911 Minutes; and newspaper article, "Officers Elected by Nurses' Association," n.d., IHS.

[41]Grace Julian Clarke, "Address on Woman's Suffrage," 1912 Minutes, Box 2, folder 1, IHS; and "Grace Julian Clarke," in *The Social Register of Indiana* (Indianapolis: The Social Register of Indiana, 1912), 45.

[42]1912 ISNA Minutes (Semi-Annual Meeting), IHS.

[43]Sandra Beth Lewenson, *Taking Charge: Nursing, Suffrage, & Feminism in America, 1873–1920* (New York: NLN Press, 1996), 185–189.

[44]Code of Ethics, Box 20, folder 9, IHS.

[45]Program, *Twenty-Fifth Annual Meeting, Indiana State Nurses Association*, 21–22 October 1927, Box 12, folder 10, IHS.

[46]1915–1918 ISNA Minutes, Box 2, folder 1, IHS.

[47]1918 ISNA Minutes, Box 2, folder 1, IHS.

[48]John Mack Faragher, et al., *Out of Many: A History of the American People, Combined Edition*, Brief 3rd ed. (Upper Saddle River, New Jersey: Prentice Hall, 2001), 231.

[49] "Official Actions of the Catholic Hospital Association with Reference to Nursing Education," Archives of the Catholic Health Association, St. Louis, Missouri.

[50]Schroder, 29–30.

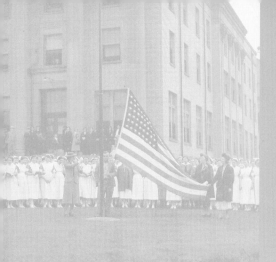

Chapter 3

"Inheritors of a Great Tradition": The Interwar Years *1920-1940*

Jane Manning, M.S.N., R.N.

"We who are nurses are inheritors of a great tradition. It is ours to guard, to strengthen, to enlarge where needed and to equip ourselves worthily for so doing."[1] These words spoken by Mary Adelaide Nutting in a tribute to Florence Nightingale in the early 1900s foretold the challenges to professional nursing organizations following World War I. The number of women in the workforce had nearly doubled since the turn of the century. By 1920 women comprised more than one-fifth of the total working population. Kalisch and Kalisch note, "It was an age of unheard of freedom for women, hard won in World War I. Women had proved they could take the place of men on countless fronts...."[2] The war also had demonstrated the effectiveness of scientific medicine and the importance of hospitals. These medical institutions began receiving an increased number of consumer-oriented, middle-class patients.

This was a time of change in many arenas in Indiana. Entertainer and banjo player Noble Sissle and other black musicians along with Hoagy Carmichael attracted large numbers of people as jazz music swept across the state. These groups spawned nightclubs where new dances such as the Charleston could be practiced. Radios and cinema brought news and entertainment to wide audiences. And the "flapper" with her lipstick, short skirt, and bobbed hair represented the new feminism.[3] While many Hoosiers working in factories and offices experienced decreased working hours, allowing them more time for leisure activities, this was not typical for nursing students. They continued to work long hours in hospitals, six to seven days a week, and then went to lectures later in the evenings.

Although a great number of women had joined nursing's ranks during the war, many student nurses dropped out of schools after the patriotic motivation wore thin. Thus, the United States faced a shortage of approximately 55,000 trained nurses in 1920.[4] Schools of nursing encountered huge recruitment

46

problems. Prospects in Indiana had grown so dire that some hospitals in smaller towns had to close their doors.

In 1921 to meet the increased demand for nurses, the ISNA and other groups conducted a recruiting campaign throughout Indiana. As reported in the *AJN*, "The Board of Directors of the Indiana State Nurses' Association recently voted to give $500 toward the fund for the student nurse recruiting campaign to be started soon." [5] During the campaign, these nurses addressed two hundred groups, including high schools, colleges, women's clubs, and teachers' institutes in an effort to interest more eligible young women in nursing. As a follow-up to this intensive effort, the ISNA appointed an Educational Committee in October 1922. Its purpose was to inform the public about the nursing profession in an attempt to keep a constant applicant flow into accredited schools of nursing, thus preventing future shortages. That same year, the Board of Examination and Registration of Nurses reported thirty-four accredited schools of nursing, with 595 applicants to enter training schools. Other campaigns for students occurred in 1924 and 1925.[6]

The ISNA continued its quest for members, increasing its membership by 31 percent by 1924. Ina M. Gaskill, president of the ISNA, described their successful strategies in a 1924 *AJN* article. Noting that other women's organizations such as the YWCA and the League of Women Voters held successful membership drives year after year, she wondered, why not the ISNA? She described a contest between the districts whereby the chair of the most successful district would be sent as a state delegate to the biennial convention, all expenses paid. Individual nurses securing the most new members were rewarded as well. Although the ISNA had a history of grass-roots organization, albeit a short one, President Gaskill concluded, "Such pulling together and teamwork had never before been shown...."[7]

ISNA Support for Child Welfare

Throughout its history, the ISNA had been instrumental in campaigns for child welfare. In 1922 the association pledged $1,000 toward the building fund of the James Whitcomb Riley Hospital for Children. The chair of the Riley Memorial Association Finance Committee wrote a thank-you letter to President Ina Gaskill. He stated, "This contribution is helping to make possible the world's greatest hospital for children and thousands of crippled and ailing children will remember those who make it possible for them to be well and strong again. It is a Good Deed."[8] The ISNA's efforts for child welfare had heightened after the passage of the 1921 Sheppard-Towner Act and the formation of the Children's Bureau. Women's groups used their recent enfranchisement to influence this federal legislation that funded educational programs in maternal and infant hygiene. In Indiana, under the direction of Dr. Ada Schweitzer, the new Division of Infant and Child Hygiene became a center for public health work in the 1920s.

Nurses in the ISNA also influenced public policy in the child welfare arena. In 1919, as a member of the State Board of Health, Dr. Schweitzer held a round-table discussion with delegates to the ISNA Annual Convention and already obtained the nurses' support for this important work by the time the Sheppard-Towner Act came into effect. By 1930 Indiana's maternal mortality rate was 6.2 deaths per 1,000 live births, an improvement over the rate of 8.1 in 1920. Even more staggering was the drop in the infant mortality rate: from 81.8 deaths per 1,000 live births in 1920 to 57.7 in 1930, largely as a result of women's work for other women and their children.[9]

The ISNA's generosity was seen in other areas. In 1922 it contributed to the American Nurses' Memorial in Bordeaux, France, in memory of the American nurses who died in World War I. In May 1924 it received a letter

Patients at City Hospital (Indianapolis) enjoying a Christmas celebration (ca. 1920s) (From the collection of the Wishard Nursing Museum)

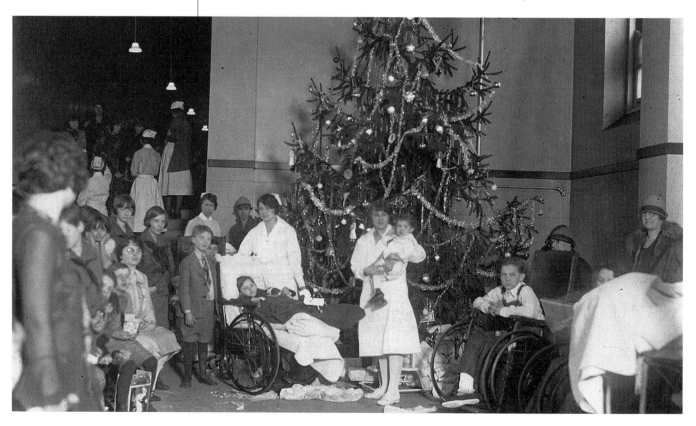

48

from Matthew O. Foley, executive secretary of the National Hospital Day Committee, thanking the association for adopting a resolution supporting National Hospital Day. "You will be interested to know that the Indiana Nurses are the first state association of which we have record which has endorsed this day and we want to congratulate you on your progressiveness in this action."[10]

Organizational Issues

At this time, membership in the ISNA consisted of registered nurses who were members of the four district associations. In 1924 this totaled 1,155 nurses. As its membership and activities increased in the early 1920s, leaders realized that volunteers could no longer handle the growing amount of office work. Thus, in 1923 the association budgeted for a part-time office worker and shared the person's time with the State Board of Examination and Registration. The two groups agreed that the ISNA would employ the person part-time as executive secretary and that the State Board would employ her the remainder of the time as educational director. Alma Scott took the dual position and began her duties in January 1924, when the ISNA established its headquarters in Indianapolis.[11]

As part of her role, Alma Scott served as chair of the State Committee on Ethical Standards. In 1928 she received an outline of basic ethical principles drawn up by the ANA Committee on Ethical Standards. She sent letters containing this proposed Code of Ethics to ISNA district chairs for their input. As district members suggested revisions, they forwarded them to the chair of the National Committee. Mrs. Scott left her ISNA position in 1929 to work for the ANA. After working her way up from other positions, she became the director of headquarters for the ANA from 1935 to 1946. An *AJN* article made several references to Mrs. Scott's Indiana roots:

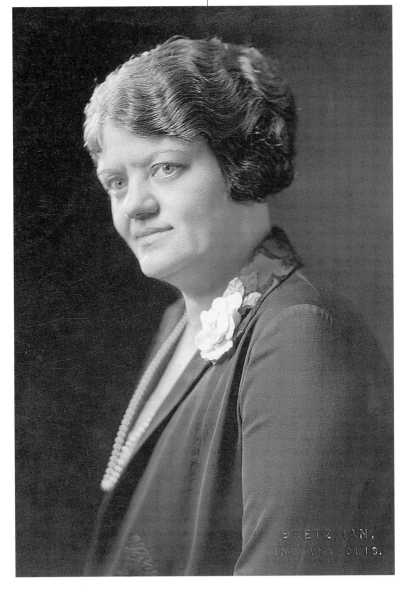

Alma Scott was ISNA executive secretary and the educational director of the Indiana State Board of Examination and Registration for Nurses. (ISNA Collection M0380, Indiana Historical Society)

Out of the Midwest and exemplifying its vigor and friendliness came Alma Ham Scott to the Headquarters of the American Nurses' Association….One of Mrs. Scott's contributions was the development of a comprehensive system of records to be used in all Indiana schools. Procedure books, so familiar in schools of nursing today, were being built up in the best schools but in many they were entirely unknown. Through her energetic work the schools were helped to organize them and to establish their use.[12]

"Cooperation Comparable to That Shown by Indiana": Nursing Education Issues

In 1924 the ISNA showed its support for the National League of Nursing Education by contributing $400 toward the organization's efforts to raise standards in schools of nursing. The editor of the *AJN* praised the Indiana association: "We have long admired the *esprit de corps* and the capacity for growth of the Indiana nurses. The program of the National League would be assured if we could all have a conception of cooperation comparable to that shown by Indiana."[13]

An ongoing concern for the ISNA involved the Nurse Practice Act. One of the association's most outstanding defenses came in 1921 when it mobilized nurses throughout the state to defeat a proposed amendment that would have lowered the state's nursing education standards. A small group of physicians operating private hospitals sponsored the amendment. Finding it difficult to get students in their small hospitals, the physicians wanted to place doctors on the State Board of Examination and Registration of Nurses, who would then try to lower the standards of the training schools. When the nurses learned that such a bill was in the making, they requested that it be held in committee until they could get organized. They demanded and received a public hearing before it came up for a second reading. Recalling the event in later years, then President Mary Meyers wrote that hundreds of nurses from across the state converged on the State House for the public hearing. The bill did not pass. Another bill, which had been presented at the 1920 ISNA Annual Convention, was introduced into the legislature instead, with the purpose of raising standards in the training schools. Passed on 19 March 1921, it increased admission requirements for students entering schools of nursing and set standards for course length. Remarking on the defeat of the original bill and the subsequent passage of the nurses' new bill, a seasoned, albeit opinionated, legislator stated that it was his first experience in the Indiana Legislature whereby a group of women worked as one team through such a long period.[14]

As in Indiana, much national attention was being given to the quality of nursing education. Nurse training was mainly by the apprenticeship method, and student nurses formed most of the hospital labor force. By the mid-1920s more than 2,000 schools of nursing existed in the United States, and the seeming scarcity of nurses during and immediately after World War I was replaced with an oversupply. Furthermore, the war and recent developments in medicine highlighted a need for changes in nursing schools and services. Begun as a classically "female" calling, nursing now demanded integration with science-based skills. Thus nursing leaders, aided by medical, hospital, educational, and lay groups, initiated several important studies.[15] One was the Goldmark Report, released to the public in 1923, calling for the establishment of schools of nursing in universities to meet the standards of other professions.

Following the Goldmark Report, in 1926 the National League for Nursing Education, the ANA, and other groups organized the Committee on the Grading of Nursing Schools. It was funded by private bequests and financial contributions of individual nurses and their associations, including the ISNA. The Grading Committee conducted a study that culminated in the 1928 publication, *Nurses, Patients and Pocketbooks*. The findings documented an oversupply of nurses, too many substandard schools, and decreasing employment opportunities. Furthermore, nearly half of the 20,000 new graduates in the country had not finished high school. The committee recommended a decrease in the number of nursing schools, higher entrance requirements, separation of nursing education and service in hospitals, and public funding for nurses' training.[16]

As the Great Depression loomed, Indiana also experienced an overproduction of nurses. Whereas trained nurses numbered 2,767 in 1920, the number had doubled by 1932. Furthermore, although Indiana had a licensing law, nurses still were not *required* to register, and other "self-styled" nurses continued to practice. A handwritten history of the ISNA reports that *Nurses, Patients and Pocketbooks* was "being studied by all nurses." One bulletin boldly noted, "EVERY INDIANA SCHOOL MUST DO ITS SHARE TO DECREASE ADMISSION OF STUDENTS." The nursing schools complied by raising admission standards. In 1932 all but one of the accredited schools raised their entrance requirements to four years of high school.[17] Also in the 1930s, some of the smaller hospital diploma programs began to close, and others started working with colleges and universities to permit nursing students to take courses there.

At this time, the ISNA and Indiana University (IU) at Bloomington joined forces to enhance nursing education. Indiana University Training School for Nurses had opened in Indianapolis in 1914, but in the 1930s courses for a baccalaureate program for RNs began at IU-Bloomington through the School of Education. At the same time, the ISNA promoted the development of a graduate education program for nurses at the university, and ISNA President Gertrude Upjohn appointed a committee to propose a curriculum. It recommended courses in administration, supervision, teaching, and public health nursing. In the summer of 1932, four nurses enrolled in the program.[18] Then in 1939, in cooperation with the ISNA and the IU School of Education, the IU Extension Division began offering classes in nursing education at seven centers. The ISNA Education Committee recommended the courses, which conferred university credit.[19]

Whereas in 1922 there were thirty-four accredited schools of nursing in the state,[20] this number had decreased to twenty-nine by 1933. Four affiliated with universities: IU Training School with Indiana University in Bloomington; Indianapolis City Hospital with Butler University; Methodist Hospital School of Nursing in Indianapolis with DePauw University, Greencastle; and Ball Memorial School of Nursing with Ball State Teachers College, Muncie. Eight nursing schools were connected with hospitals with fewer than 100 beds.[21] Efforts to improve education did not succeed in all areas. Indiana ranked twenty-third in the nation with respect to reasonable working hours for its students. While the State Board of Examination of Nurses handled many of these matters, ISNA President Lulu Cline reiterated one of the ISNA's major goals when she emphasized to her fellow members in 1933, "You are indirectly a part of the State Board of Nursing Education and it needs you to *help mold the opinions* of those who are responsible for education of nurses" [italics added for emphasis].[22]

Black women still faced limited educational opportunities. In the 1930s Indianapolis City Hospital School of Nursing admitted black students, but only on a quota basis. Although all students had classes and ate together, black students had to live on a separate floor and could not participate in social activities in the nurses' residence.[23]

By the mid-1930s, in order to have a nurse training school, hospitals had to provide a variety of services and have adequate finances to be qualified to give thorough training. This included having a minimum of twenty-five beds. The greatest trouble came from small hospitals owned and managed by physicians. An ISNA member recalled one doctor in Madison, Indiana, who conducted a nursing school in a ten-bed facility. To meet state requirements, he brought in fifteen additional beds and stored them in the attic, thus meeting the criterion of twenty-five beds![24]

Networking between the ISNA and the American Red Cross continued in the 1930s. In 1933, for example, an amendment to the Indiana Nurse Practice Act had been presented to the state legislature. It was designed to take authority away from the State Board of Examination and Registration of Nurses and enable hospitals with a daily census of only twelve patients to conduct schools of nursing. This, of course, would have lowered standards, and Executive Secretary Helen Teal appealed to Mrs. Adelbert Flynn, chair of the Red Cross

ISNA members attending the biennial Meeting of the Members in Fort Wayne (1934). Left to right: Helen Teal (ISNA executive director 1931–47), Delta Schmoe, Mary Walsh, person unidentified, and Mary McDonald Van Sweringen. (ISNA Collection M0380, Indiana Historical Society)

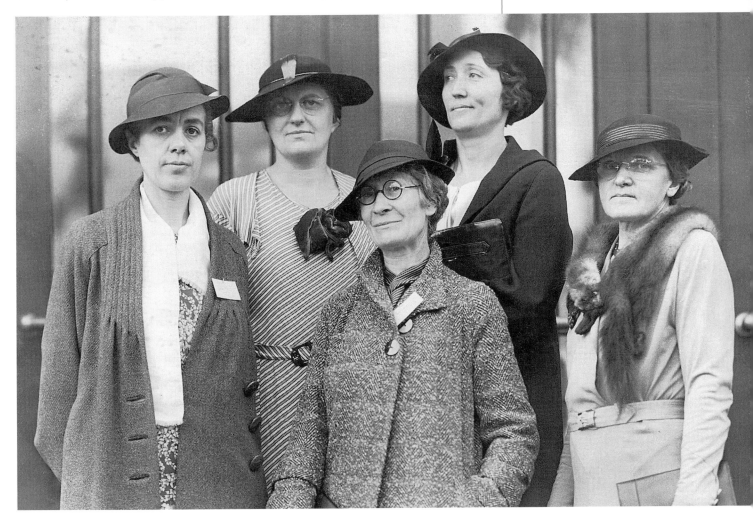

Cass County Chapter, for help. Learning that graduates from such schools would not be eligible for enrollment in the American Red Cross Nursing Service, Mrs. Flynn, also vice chairman of the State Democratic Party, helped defeat the amendment. Indeed, it died in committee. The *AJN* heralded, "The Red Cross has marshaled its forces and assisted in many types of disasters, but this…is the first time that the standards of nursing in a given state have been saved because an individual possessing knowledge of Red Cross affairs recognized the danger and proceeded promptly to the rescue."[25]

Problems with Unemployment

The Great Depression was the worst economic crisis in American history, and by 1933 one-fourth of the nation's labor force was jobless. As conditions worsened, the ISNA began concentrating on finding work for graduates. In the 1930s, most graduate nurses worked in patients' homes as private duty nurses. The demand for their services had been decreasing since the early 1920s, however, as more patients entered hospitals for care. At that time, the ISNA had established a Private Duty section to help solve the problem. The association also contributed to the ANA Relief Fund (established in 1911) for nurses who could no longer work.

Beginning in 1927 the ISNA became a member of the Midwest Division of the ANA, in conjunction with the state associations of Illinois, Wisconsin, Iowa, and Michigan. This division was established to deal with local problems, and it held meetings biennially in the spring between ANA conventions. One of the division's most important committees was the Committee on the Distribution of Nursing Service. Finding qualified nurses for various positions was becoming increasingly more difficult because nurses were more mobile. Furthermore, employers sought nurses with extra preparation in education and public health. As the Great Depression brought widespread unemployment, the committee worked to facilitate sharing of available nursing opportunities. In addition the committee: 1) sent letters to superintendents of those hospitals without nursing students to hire only graduate nurses registered in Indiana; 2) approached the Indiana State Medical Association and Indiana Catholic Hospital Association to encourage them to employ Indiana RNs in preference to practical nurses in hourly nursing service; and 3) put an editorial in the *Indiana State Medical Journal* urging the employment of Indiana RNs. These efforts proved successful. In some districts, private duty nurses decreased their individual working hours from twenty to eight or twelve hours, thus sharing the workload with others. In hospitals without student nurses, employment of graduate nurses increased 49 percent between 1932 and 1933, and practical nurses decreased by a third.[26]

In the 1930s even fewer patients could afford private duty, and it was during this time that graduate nurses began to move into hospitals for employment. In 1930, nursing leader Janet Geister reported to the 27th National Biennial Nursing Convention, "The steadily increasing number of graduates securing employment in hospitals are the most hopeful signs to both patient and nurse."[27] That graduate nurses could give the best nursing care became the rationale for their move into the hospital workforce. Still, as general staff nurses, women worked for very low salaries, sometimes thirty dollars to fifty dollars a month.[28]

In an effort to help the unemployed, the United States Congress passed the National Industrial Recovery Act in 1933 as part of legislation under the New Deal. However, the law did not apply to unemployed nurses. Responding to the implications for the profession, the ANA issued position statements that addressed the need for an economic recovery plan that considered the thousands of unemployed graduate nurses. This plan included considering nurses' salaries and endorsing eight-hour shifts, while still allowing for the best care for patients.[29] In their *History of Nursing*, Stewart and Austin note, "The eight-hour day in nursing services became more general after it had been tried as a device to spread the work during the period of acute unemployment. These and other problems led to closer relationships among nurses in various fields and among members of the medical and health professions generally."[30]

Another aspect of New Deal legislation came in 1933 when the federal government authorized the creation of the Civil Works Administration (CWA) that provided jobs and wages to those able to work. It helped nurses and the general public by providing funds for bedside nursing care in the homes of unemployment relief recipients, under the supervision of the State Bureau of Public Health Nursing. Executive Secretary Helen Teal was a member of the Advisory Committee on Nursing for the CWA's Indiana Commission. In December 1933, she sent letters to the ISNA members describing CWA nursing positions that included "public health nursing, immunization programs, dental caries survey sponsored by the Dental Society, staff duty nursing in hospitals and clinics, and nursing service in orphanages."[31] These were short-term nursing tasks wherein less experienced nurses could be guided by advisory nurses. The CWA was an emergency measure, and President Roosevelt dismantled the program in the spring of 1934 after it had helped people weather the winter months. Through the CWA, 414 Indiana nurses obtained work in institutions and especially in public health projects. Nurses made 17,638 visits to nearly 6,000 patients. Helen Teal listed six additional benefits: 1) the ratio of public health nurses for the urban population went from 1: 9,148 to 1: 3,579 and for the rural population 1: 42,936 to 1: 9,116; 2) medical societies in most counties that had CWA nurses approved standing orders, which helped nurses and protected patients; 3) a plan had been created for adequate public health nursing supervision at the local and state level; 4) communities realized what nurses could do in a public health program; 5) many CWA nurses inquired about further preparation to better qualify themselves for Indiana positions; and 6) health commissioners had a new vision of how effective nurses could be in their programs.[32]

After the CWA's demise, Indiana's Advisory Committee on Nursing for the CWA had been told provisionally that statewide public health nursing projects might be continued indefinitely, if the committee so recommended, through another New Deal program, the Emergency Relief Administration (ERA). To extend the public health nursing project was problematic, however, because young graduate nurses with meager experience and no specialized public health training had been utilized, relief wages were adequate only if one could live with relatives, and there were minimum standards of qualifications for the nurses. Also pertinent were the sporadic accusations by representatives of the medical association of poor technique and ethics made against public health nurses. Thus, ISNA directors replied that only nurses schooled in public health nursing should be appointed to public health positions and requested the medical association's cooperation in upholding these standards.[33]

The Advisory Committee on Nursing recommended continuing the nursing public health programs, but it stipulated that civil sponsors should pay for nurses' travel and supplies, and in turn, nurses should take regional educational institutes on rural nursing. At the end of 1934 the ERA employed 150 nurses, and the education project involved cooperation with the ISNA, State Board of Public Health Nursing, American Red Cross, State Division of Public Health, Indiana State Tuberculosis Association, Women's Work Division of the ERA, and the State Board of Nurse Examiners.[34]

Public health and private duty nursing issues remained prevalent in the 1930s. For example, at the 1931 ISNA convention in Gary, Ella Best, field secretary for the ANA, presented a paper about registry development and then attended a breakfast where private duty nurses could discuss their problems with her.[35] At the 1934 convention, the Public Health Section held a meeting to discuss whether the ISNA should seek legislation legalizing and protecting public health nursing. At that same convention, the Private Duty Section heard Ethel Swope, a representative from the ANA, "who gave a stirring address urg-

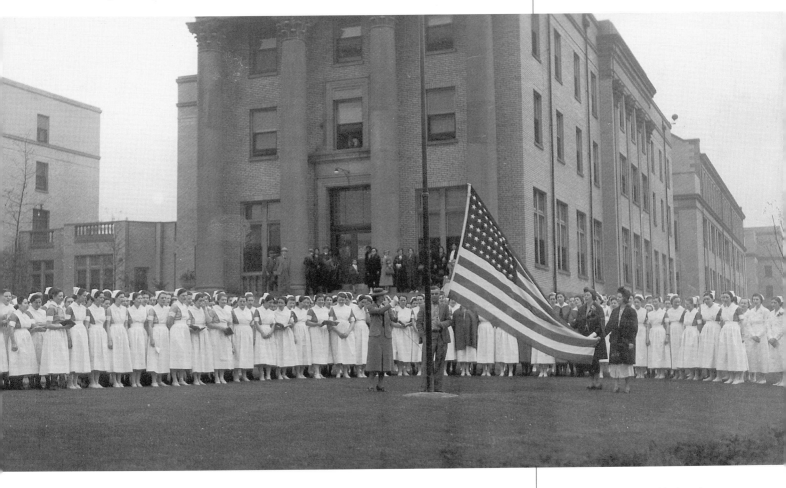

ing the Indiana nurses to strive for an eight-hour day."[36] Thus, in 1935 ISNA member Delta Schmoe wrote, "In order to provide a better nursing service and be able to give quality nursing to our patients, the Northeast District of ISNA decided to adopt eight hours as a reasonable working day for private duty nurses." Fees were four dollars for eight hours and six dollars for twelve hours.[37]

Other highlights in the 1930s included: 1) the establishment of the ISNA headquarters at the Circle Tower Building in downtown Indianapolis in 1930; 2) the increase in the number of districts from four to nine in 1934; and 3) the first publication of the *Lamp* in July 1937. *The Lamp* was the official bulletin of the ISNA and continued until April 1951 at which time it became the *Indiana Nurse*. As the association made its mark in improving the nursing profession and in

May 12, 1937, was National Hospital Day. The American Legion Auxiliary conducted a flag ceremony in Indianapolis. (From the collection of the Wishard Nursing Museum)

working for nurses, its membership grew from 1,711 members in 1930 to 3,544 in 1940.[38] At the 1940 joint meeting of the ISNA and the Indiana State League of Nursing Education, 606 nurses attended, including 97 students.[39]

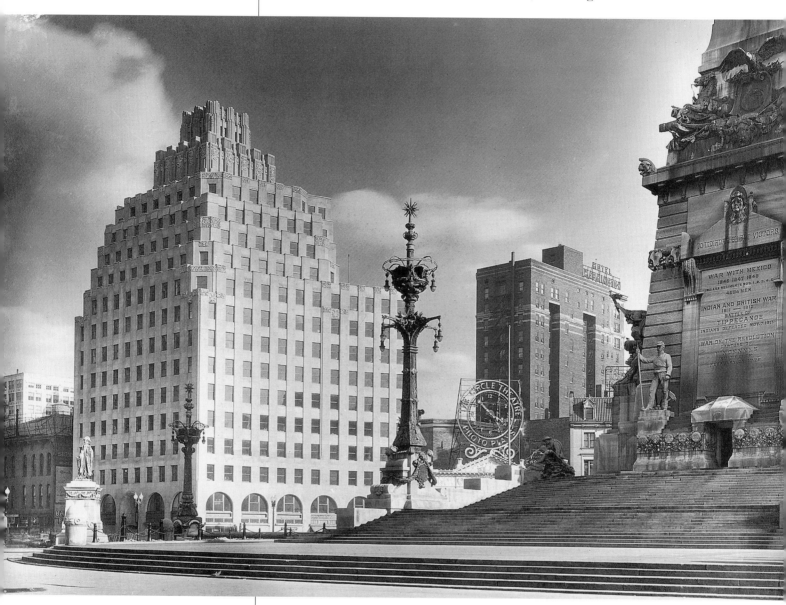

ISNA's offices were first located in the Circle Tower (Indianapolis). The offices, on the twelfth floor of the pyramid-shaped building, served as the headquarters through March 1951. (ISNA Collection M0380, Indiana Historical Society)

Endnotes

[1]Isabel M. Stewart and Anne L. Austin, *A History of Nursing* (New York: G.P. Putnam's Sons, 1962), taken from a tribute to Florence Nightingale in the dedication section.

[2]Philip A. Kalisch and Beatrice J. Kalisch, *The Advance of American Nursing, 3rd edition* (J. B. Lippincott Company, 1995), 239.

[3]James H. Madison, *Indiana through Tradition and Change: A History of the Hoosier State and Its People, 1920–1945* (Indianapolis: Indiana Historical Society, 1982), 364–365.

[4]Kalisch and Kalisch, 240.

[5]"Nursing News and Announcements," *AJN* 21 (1921): 742.

[6]*Report of the State Board of Registration and Examination of Nurses for the State of Indiana, for the Year Ending Sept. 30, 1922* (Indianapolis: Wm. B. Burford, 1923); Alma H. Scott, typed copy of "Indiana State Nurses Association," 1925, Box 12, folder 9; and 1926, Box 12, folder 10, IHS.

[7]"A Membership Campaign," *AJN* 24, no. 13 (1924): 1,023–1,025.

[8]L. C. Huesmann to Ina M. Gaskill, 4 December 1922, Box 11, folder 1, IHS.

[9]Madison, 321–322.

[10]Matthew O. Foley to June Gray, 6 May 1924, Box 11, folder 1, IHS.

[11]Mary M. Schroder, "History of the Indiana State Nurses' Association" (M.A. thesis, University of Chicago, 1958), 38.

[12]Ethel P. Clarke, "Alma Ham Scott—Organizer," *AJN* 36, no. 2 (1936): 149–152.

[13]"Editorials," *AJN* 24 (1924): 191.

[14]Schroder, 36–38.

[15]Stewart and Austin, 215.

[16]Susan M. Reverby, *Ordered to Care: The Dilemma of American Nursing, 1850–1945* (New York and Cambridge: Cambridge University Press, 1987), 170–171.

[17]"Salient Facts for Ready Reference," Box 26, Folder 2, IHS.

[18]Ann Marriner-Tomey, ed., *Nursing at Indiana University: 75 Years at the Heart of Health Care* (Indianapolis: Indianapolis University School of Nursing, 1989), 5, 57.

[19]"News," *AJN* 39, no. 11 (1939): 1,278.

[20]"Report of the State Board of Registration and Examination of Nurses of the State of Indiana," 30 September 1922, Box 26, folder 2.

[21]Dotaline E. Allen, *History of Nursing in Indiana* (Indianapolis: Wolfe Publishing Co., 1950), 62.

[22]L. V. Cline, "The Present Problems and Needs of Indiana," October 1933, Box 3, folder 12, IHS.

[23]Hester Anne Hale, *Caring for the Community: The History of Wishard Hospital* (Indianapolis: Wishard Memorial Foundation, 1999), 76.

[24]Elizabeth Johnson, Memo Book, 1937, Box 12, folder 10, IHS.

[25]"Red Cross to the Rescue," *AJN* 33, no. 3 (1933): 228.

[26]"Report of Chairman of Committee on Distribution of Nursing Service and Registries," 15 October 1933, Box 3, folder 12, IHS.

[27]Nora Tudor, "Minutes of the 27th National Biennial Nursing Convention," Box 12, folder 10, IHS.

[28]Allen, 62–63.

[29]Karen J. Egenes and Wendy K. Burgess, *Faithfully Yours: A History of Nursing in Illinois* (Chicago: Illinois Nurses' Association, 2001), 78.

[30]Stewart and Austin, 219.

[31]Helen Teal to Miss Smith, 6 December 1933, Box 10, folder 13, IHS.

[32]Helen Teal, "What Was Accomplished in Public Health by CWA Nurses in Indiana," 1934; and "Final Report of CWA Nurses in Public Health," 1934, Box 10, folder 13, IHS.

[33]Helen Teal, "Indiana's ERA Nursing Institutes," *AJN* 34, no. 12 (December 1934): 1,158; and Advisory Committee on Nursing to Letitia Carter, Director, Women's Work, ERA, Box 10, folder 13.

[34]Ibid.

[35]"News," *AJN* 31, no. 12 (1931): 1,455.

[36]Minutes, ISNA Annual Convention, 2 October 1934, Box 4, folder 1, IHS.

[37]Delta Schmoe, document from the Nursing Service Bureau, 15 April 1935, Box 11, folder 1, IHS.

[38]*The Lamp* 4, no. 3 (November 1940): 4.

[39]"News About Nursing," *AJN* 40, no. 12 (1940): 1,428.

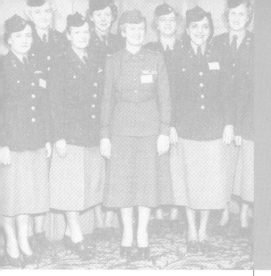

Chapter 4

"Service to Country and the Profession": World War II and Professional Growth *1940-1960*

Diane Eaton, M.S.N., R.N.

During her welcoming remarks at the 1940 ISNA Annual Convention, Southwest District President Susan Shoemaker reflected how appropriate it was that nurses were meeting in Evansville, the same city where Clara Barton came in 1884 to care for flood victims. Once again, Indiana nurses were preparing for a national crisis. World War II seemed inevitable, and nurses were aware of the impact the European war eventually would have on the need for their services.

The language of service to country and humankind was a familiar one to Mrs. Shoemaker and the ISNA members. Her reference to nurses "banding together as a unit for national service"[1] was a theme spoken throughout the 1940s. Presentations that reflected the moral and patriotic sentiments of the decade were sprinkled throughout annual conventions and publications. Programs also revealed nursing's traditional links to religion. Members sang "God Bless America" and recited the Lord's Prayer. At the 1940 Annual Convention, Sister Theresa from St. Mary's Hospital, Evansville, gave the invocation, and she focused on ideals of loyalty to God, justice to those served, fortitude in the face of danger, and charity so that no person would be turned away because of poverty.[2]

President Anne Dugan continued the religious, patriotic, and service themes in her opening remarks at the 1941 Annual Convention: "And, because of the anxiety of the times, we feel more than ever the bonds that hold us together, the bonds of human service....With Christ we journey, and we walk with our footsteps in his footprints; it is He who is our guide and the burning flame that illuminates our path."[3]

As the nation came out of the throes of the Great Depression, economic security continued to be an issue for the ISNA. Its Committee of Relief and Service was active throughout the early 1940s, making loans to those members with critical needs and reporting this information at each of the annual conventions.[4]

The Harmon Plan for Nurses, a national annuity plan started in 1929, was offered to the ISNA members in the 1940s as a means for economic protection against sickness, accident, and retirement.[5] Economic security rose to a more complex level following World War II with the introduction of employee health care benefits. Most hospitals, however, did not offer this to nurses, leading the ISNA to focus attention on updating personnel polices in the workplace. Another growing awareness was the need for professional liability insurance, which Maginnis and Associates offered to all members beginning in 1953. Especially significant to the ISNA members in the 1940s and 1950s was the economic threat posed by auxiliary workers, an issue to be examined later in this chapter.

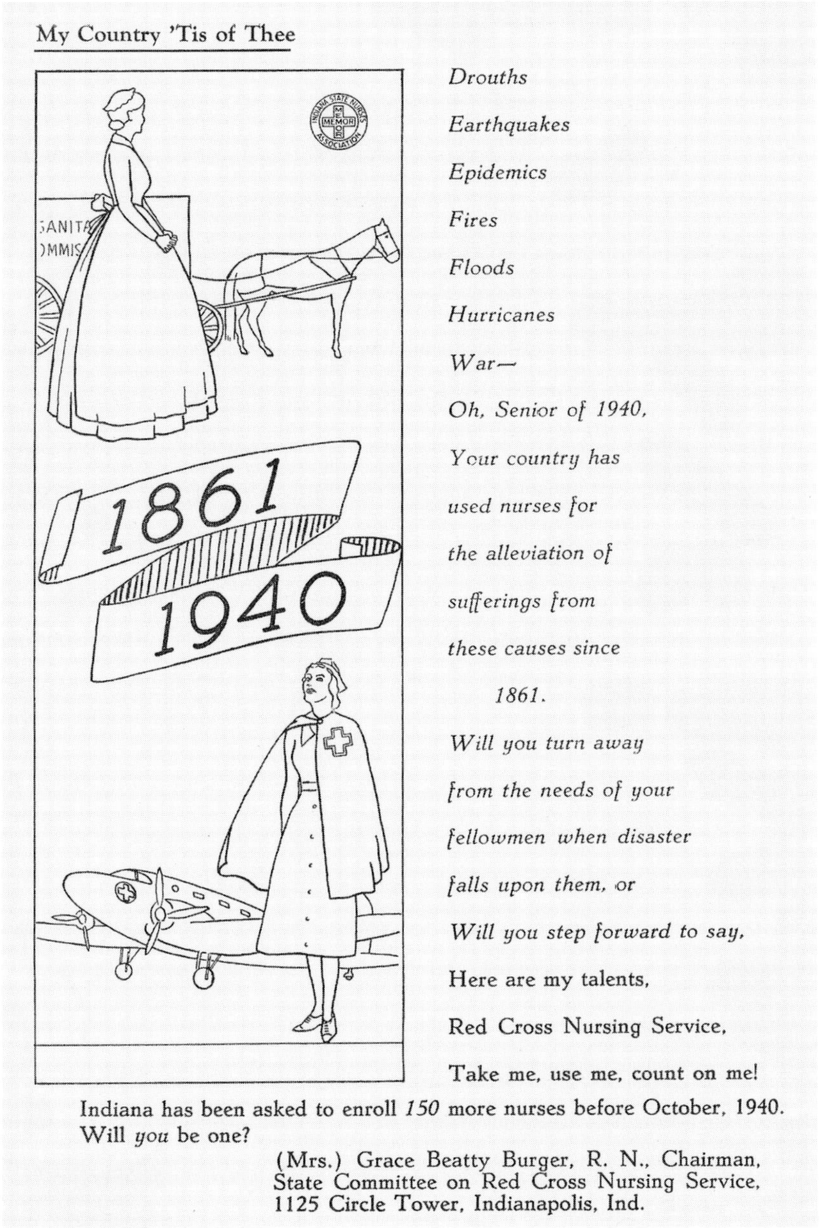

My Country 'Tis of Thee

Drouths

Earthquakes

Epidemics

Fires

Floods

Hurricanes

War—

Oh, Senior of 1940,

Your country has

used nurses for

the alleviation of

sufferings from

these causes since

1861.

Will you turn away

from the needs of your

fellowmen when disaster

falls upon them, or

Will you step forward to say,

Here are my talents,

Red Cross Nursing Service,

Take me, use me, count on me!

Indiana has been asked to enroll *150* more nurses before October, 1940. Will *you* be one?

(Mrs.) Grace Beatty Burger, R. N., Chairman, State Committee on Red Cross Nursing Service, 1125 Circle Tower, Indianapolis, Ind.

ISNA was actively involved with recruiting for the Red Cross Nursing Service. This 1940 ad indicated that Indiana was asked to sign up 150 additional nurses for the service. (*The Lamp*, ISNA Archives)

"America Needs You": The World War II Years

Whereas in the 1930s many nurses were pleading for jobs, their employment opportunities expanded during World War II. Prior to America's entrance into the war, the Indiana State Board of Health contacted the ISNA to establish a committee to address the military's growing nursing needs. In June 1941 the ISNA set up the Nursing Council for War Services, led by President Anne Dugan, Executive Secretary Helen Teal, and representatives from each district and the Indiana State Board of Health. To procure enough military nurses, the Council worked with the districts to organize local nursing war councils in every county. The workload was so time-consuming that a separate office with a full-time clerk and part-time nurse was established and remained active until 1946.[6]

During the war years, the ISNA focused most of its work on the Nursing War Council's tasks of mobilizing and educating nurses. Each local council sent postcards to nurses in their counties to inform them about the war efforts. They established a "Nurse Power File" on each nurse that recorded the nurse's school, license number, last active nursing employment, any special preparation such as surgical experience, availability for emergency duty, and the number and ages of children.[7] This information could then be used to contact inactive nurses who could replace those assigned to military duty. To get the inactive nurses ready for reassignments, the ISNA developed a refresher course and a self-study review course for those who could not attend the teacher-led program.

"America Needs You" was the theme of ISNA's 1942 Annual Convention, and afterward, the association collaborated with many organizations to meet the country's nursing needs.[8] Indiana was assigned a quota of 910 nurses for the Red Cross's First Reserve Nursing Service, to be reached by 1 October 1942, and 80 nurses a month to be furnished to the Armed Forces. To speed up nurses' availability for military service, the ISNA persuaded the Indiana State Board to increase its administration of licensure examinations from two times a year to three.[9] The great demand for wartime nurses was alleviated somewhat in 1943 when the Cadet Nurse Corps formed. Sponsored by the U.S. Public Health Service, the program subsidized nursing students' entire education. Many Indiana nurses took advantage of this offer. In the mid-1940s, for example, almost all of Indianapolis City Hospital's students were enrolled in the Cadet Nurse Corps program.[10]

In 1943 because of gasoline shortages, the U.S. Office of Defense Transportation discouraged conventions if long-distance transportation was necessary. Thus, that year the ISNA Board of Directors recommended that annual meetings be suspended throughout the duration of the war and for six months following. The elected officers transacted organizational business in written reports and through personal contacts.[11] In preparation for the meeting suspensions, the leadership challenged each district to work on nursing student recruitment and to find new methods to inform members about nursing issues.[12]

"Recruitment Committee of One"

In addition to the war effort, the ISNA still pursued its goal of improving educational standards in nursing schools. In Indiana, as in the rest of the country, nursing service and education existed within the hospital setting. Hospitals underwrote the cost of nurses' education and housing through students' apprenticeship training or clinical work. In 1940 the educational director, Mary T. Walsh, visited all twenty-eight nursing schools in the state and reported that progress was being made to raise the educational standards.[13] In the same year, the ISNA's Committee on Post-Graduate Study and Education, which acted as a liaison between schools and the ISNA, recommended that alumnae associations create scholarships to assist head nurses, nursing supervisors, and instructors in obtaining advanced training.[14]

In 1942 ISNA President Anne Dugan encouraged everyone to be a "committee of one" to recruit women into nursing programs. Her suggestions for the districts included letter writing; talks to clubs, business groups, churches, schools, and PTAs; and alumnae-sponsored teas for high school students.[15] The need for nurses was so great that the ISNA press release from the 1942 convention read: "Nurses who are married or in the over 40 age group should return to civilian staffs for part time or full time work, thereby releasing nurses who can serve with the military."[16] In 1943 the ISNA produced a promotional tape titled *Hidden Nurses* to increase women's awareness of nurses' important roles during the war years. Mrs. Latys Benning Stewart wrote the audio portion and gave speaking roles to Captain Mary Walker of the Army Nurse Corps and Miss Isabel Maitland Stewart of Columbia University. Through its many efforts, the ISNA was able to fulfill 1,515 military positions by 1946.[17]

During and after the war, the demand for nurses at home continued in hospitals and industry. In 1946 the ANA formed the Professional Counseling and

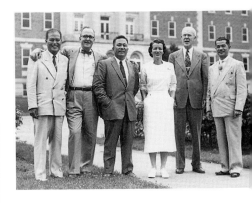

Helen Johnson (center), with Veterans Administration officials, became chief of nursing services at Veterans Administration Hospitals, Fort Benjamin Harrison and Indianapolis, in 1952. She served as ISNA president 1950–52.

Placement Service (PC&PS).[18] The PC&PS counselors traveled across the state meeting with the ISNA districts, high school students, and student nurses to inform them of the many opportunities in nursing. Interested applicants placed a professional biography with the service, which then contacted them when an employer filed a position that met their qualifications.[19]

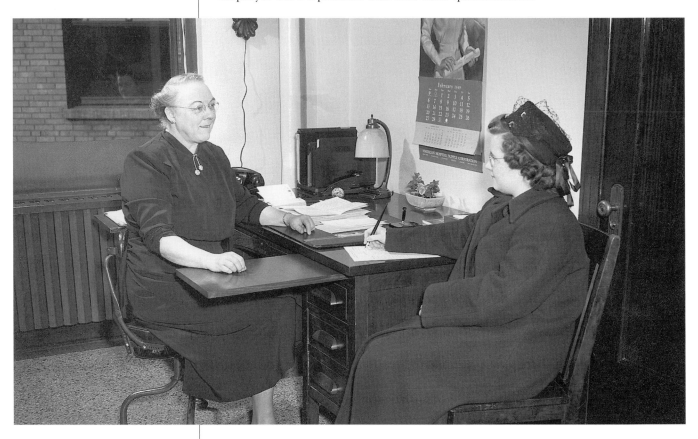

Edwina MacDougall (left) served as the first director of ISNA's Professional Counseling and Placement Service 1946–56. This service assisted many new nursing graduates. In 1949 MacDougall spoke with applicant Thelma Brooks. (ISNA Collection M0380, Indiana Historical Society)

"And they should wear colored uniforms":
Managing Auxiliary Personnel

Postwar economic growth brought great opportunities for women, who gained jobs in nursing, teaching, and other fields. Between 1940 and 1950, the number of nurses increased by 28.1 percent. While the greatest number of women remained in the traditional areas of service, things were beginning to change. After 1950 women's enrollment in nursing schools decreased by 50 percent as more women entered the fields of engineering, sales, and other areas.[20]

Thus, the postwar years began with a critical nursing shortage all over the country, especially in hospitals. The Hill-Burton Act of 1946 had resulted in an increase of hospital beds. More people were using hospitals because of biomedical and surgical advances; the expansion of private insurance plans; and the wide availability of penicillin, sulfa drugs, and streptomycin that drastically reduced hospital infections. In addition, the U.S. birth rate had soared, and more mothers were delivering their babies in hospitals. Increased marriages resulted in women leaving the workforce altogether to care for families at home. Inside the hospital, professional nurses moved farther from the bedside as they had to take on more administrative duties, leaving patient care in the hands of students, nursing assistants, and other auxiliary personnel.[21]

After the war, professional nursing organizations took a decisive stand on the use of auxiliary workers. Education and accreditation of auxiliary workers in the form of practical nurses was at the top of the ISNA's discussion list in 1947. While leaders accepted the need for additional nurses in the form of auxiliary personnel, they asserted prerogatives over their education. At the 1947 Annual Convention, President E. Nancy Scramlin stated, "Auxiliary workers are already trained on the job in many of our hospitals. The question is not, therefore, shall a second level nurse be trained, but shall ISNA take a leadership in the establishment of definite schools with a definite curriculum." Following nursing leaders across the country, the ISNA took the stand that professional nurses should direct the education of auxiliary personnel. President Scramlin justified this by referring members back to their articles of incorporation, which stated that "the object of this Association shall be...the furtherance of the efficient and scientific care of the sick."[22]

The House of Delegates approved a motion to form a Committee on Practical Nursing. Along with the Indiana State Board of Nurses, they worked to establish schools of practical nursing. To maintain control over this new division of labor, the State Board agreed to continue working with the ISNA on planning the curriculum if licensure was part of the process.[23]

Private-duty nurses especially felt threatened by auxiliary workers. At the 1947 Private Duty Section meeting, members made several recommendations to the ISNA board about the future of practical nurses. Reflecting their need to protect the registered nurse's standing, these included: that there was a place for practical nurses within the health care arena; that practical nurses should have a definite curriculum with a major focus being the patient and his or her surroundings; that the administration of drugs and giving treatments should be of minimum importance in their curriculum; that the public should be able to differentiate between private-duty nurses and practical nurses; and that they wear a colored uniform rather than a white one.[24] In this way, members looked for a way to distinguish between the outward appearance of RNs and practical nurses.

The 1948 Annual Convention gave considerable attention to the issue of auxiliary nurses. President Leona Adams addressed members' anxieties about the coming of this new worker with these words:

> *Are we afraid she will take away the things we have long felt the prerogative of the professional nurse?....Are we afraid the Practical Nurse will take our jobs away from us?....There is not much question as to whether or not we WILL move—for if we do not take some action to supplement professional nursing care with that of other trained workers, there are groups ready to step in and take the matter out of our hands.*[25]

In addition, Hilda M. Torrop, director of the Michigan Practical Nurse Project, spoke about the characteristics of a practical nurse:

> *A thumbnail sketch of the practical nurse student shows a man or woman between the ages of 18 and 50 who have completed the elementary school or various high school terms....Because practical nurses live so long and closely with patients, such matters as personal appearance, grammar, table manners and interests outside of nursing are extremely important. The same assets that make for success in any field are sought when enrolling a practical nurse: student ability to get along with people, honesty, vitality of purpose, teachability, dependability, and most important, acceptance of bedside nursing as a career.*[26]

Miss Torrop's speech reflected the sentiments of nursing leaders who sought to limit the scope of the practical nurse's work to exclude management roles.

Following Miss Torrop's speech was a report by a special committee of the ISNA and Indiana State Board members, which had formed a year earlier to study the problem. This joint committee consisted of Caroline Hauerstein; E. Nancy Scramlin from the ISNA; and Hortense Hurst, state supervisor for the Home Economics Education and Vocational Division, State Department of Public Instruction. Based on their survey of practical nurse training schools in Michigan and Illinois, they recommended the following: 1) that Indiana develop a statewide curriculum committee; 2) that the committee reassess its plan to locate programs in rural areas due to the expense of running schools with minimum resources; 3) that a conference committee be established to work through multiple issues involved in establishing a practical school of nursing; and 4) that practical nurses take a certification examination.[27]

In 1949 after input from the districts and the ANA, the ISNA Board of Directors agreed to use the term Licensed Practical Nurse (LPN) in the Nurse Practice bill. They lobbied the legislature to pass the bill for state licensure of the LPN, and the governor signed it into law on 8 March 1949.

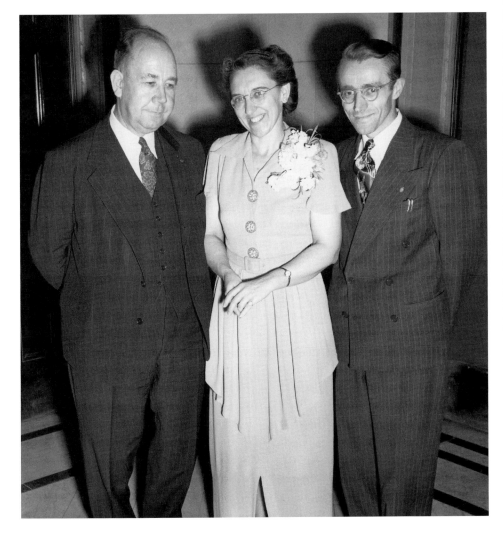

In 1948 ISNA President Leona Adams met with Indiana State Senators Maehling (left) and Baran. (ISNA Collection M0380, Indiana Historical Society)

The ISNA at Mid-Century

In 1948 credentials for registered nurses became more restrictive. The nursing profession responded to the critical nursing shortage by instituting aggressive school accreditation programs and launching national studies. At that time, the dichotomy between collegiate and diploma programs, which educated 90 percent of nursing students, became more pronounced. Several events occurred that stimulated the ISNA's activities in education. The first was the 1948 Brown Report, which indicated the future direction that professional organizations such as the ISNA would take. The Brown Report revealed that the majority of American nursing schools still trained by the apprenticeship method, and it recommended that professional education should occur at the university level. Hospital programs could exist in the interim to meet urgent nursing demands, but diploma schools had no place in nursing's future. The Brown Report advocated a more rigid division of labor between professional nurses educated at the baccalaureate level and technical nurses trained in diploma schools. The baccalaureate nurses would supervise the technical nurses and LPNs, an issue that set off a controversy that would not end for decades.[28]

The Brown Report galvanized the ISNA and other groups of health care professionals. Under the auspices of the ISNA, the Indiana State League of Nursing Education, and the Indiana State Board of Nurses, a joint Committee for the Improvement of Nursing in Indiana was formed. The committee hired Dr. Genevieve R. Bixler, a nationally recognized research consultant, and two associates to conduct a survey of all the state's nursing schools. Dr. Bixler presented the findings at the 1952 ISNA Convention, concluding that "facilities for nursing education in Indiana must be improved, possibly by consolidating, with all schools ultimately accredited nationally and all programs on a level of instruction comparable to that of colleges if the state is to be able to produce the kind of nurse the public requires."[29]

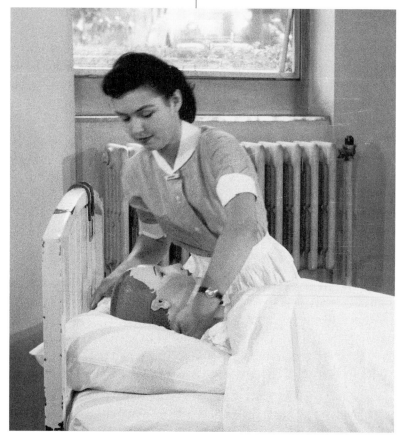

Nursing student practiced skills on a simulated model in 1949. (ISNA Collection M0380, Indiana Historical Society)

In 1947 before the Brown Report came out, Indiana University had started a program leading to the Master of Science in Education with a major in nursing education. Soon thereafter, baccalaureate programs were started in Goshen College and Evansville College. By 1950 six Indiana schools of nursing interchanged with colleges or universities leading to the baccalaureate degree. For example, Saint Mary's School of Nursing, run by the Sisters of the Holy Cross, had opened in 1936, and by 1948 it offered a five-year program leading to the Bachelor of Science in Nursing. The clinical experience was provided in the sisters' hospital in Columbus, Ohio. Similarly, in 1950 the Indiana State Teachers College began a four-year program leading to a Bachelor of Science in Nursing. Students took theoretical courses the first year at Indiana State and then spent three years in association with Terre Haute's Union Hospital where they earned a diploma in nursing. In 1954 DePauw University began one of the first four-year baccalaureate programs in the state. At the same time, small diploma schools continued to close so that by 1962 Indiana had only twenty-three schools of nursing: seventeen hospital diploma schools, four baccalaureate programs, and two associate degree programs. This was a decrease of 39.5 percent since 1908.[30]

Collaborative alliances such as the one forming the Committee for the Improvement in Nursing Education had long been the ISNA's strong point. In her Presidential Address of 20 March 1947, E. Nancy Scramlin foresaw the importance of alliances and collaborative efforts for ISNA's future:

> *Many of the changes that involve nursing are the inevitable part of the global post-war problems. America has learned…that no nation can remain isolated from the world and its problems. Professions and individuals must also learn that survival depends upon sharing of responsibilities and working together for common goals. So, the problems of nursing—economic, auxiliary workers, education and even the controversial Structure Study are all a part of the larger struggle of earnest people endeavoring to find better techniques of living together—in order that there shall be a maximum of good living with a minimum of want and friction.[31]*

In 1947, E. Nancy Scramlin resigned the presidency to become the ISNA's executive secretary. She held that position from 1947-59.

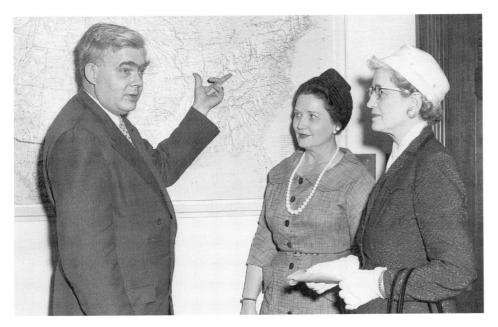

ISNA President Genevieve Beghtel and Executive Secretary E. Nancy Scramlin met with U.S. Representative Charles Brownson at the 1958 American Nurses Association Legislative Conference in Washington, D.C. (ISNA Collection M0380, Indiana Historical Society)

In the 1940s and 1950s the ISNA was actively involved in several alliances. Members worked with the Indiana League for Nursing; Health Council for the State Board of Health; Inter-professional Health Council; Medical Care Committee for the Department of Public Welfare; and the Indiana Follow-up Committee of the White House Conference on Children. The association also formed a joint committee with the Indiana Hospital Association to study the problems confronting both associations from the standpoint of standardizing technologies, personnel policies, and practices.

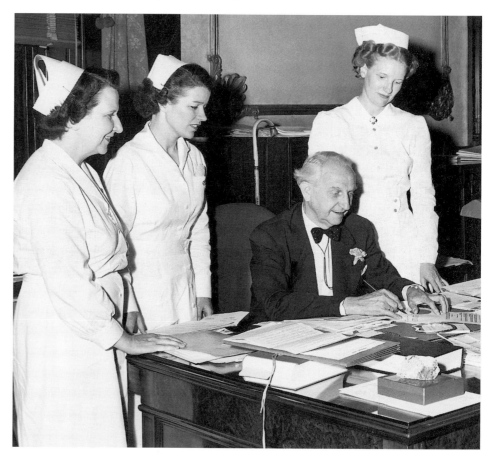

Members of ISNA committees met with Governor Henry Shricker in 1951 at the Indiana Statehouse. Pictured are (L to R): Anne Dugan, chairman, Civil Defense Committee; Helen Johnson, ISNA president; and Mary Ellen Lutz, chairman, Public Relations Committee. (ISNA Collection M0380, Indiana Historical Society)

Organizational Changes:
Districts, the Lifeblood of the Association

Growth of the ISNA came through the work of each district. By 1940 the state's nine districts showed a total membership of 3,544. Between 1943 and 1946 while the annual meetings were suspended, districts continued to have local meetings, programs, and membership drives. In the 1940s and 1950s several new districts formed, and district size became a recurring theme. Discussion of redistricting centered on the loss of members in larger districts due to greater travel time to meetings, while smaller districts grew.[32] In 1946 the ANA no longer demanded that a nurse be a member of the alumnae association, and the ISNA changed its bylaws. From then on, a nurse had only to join the district association of her place of residence, making her an automatic member of the ISNA and the ANA.[33]

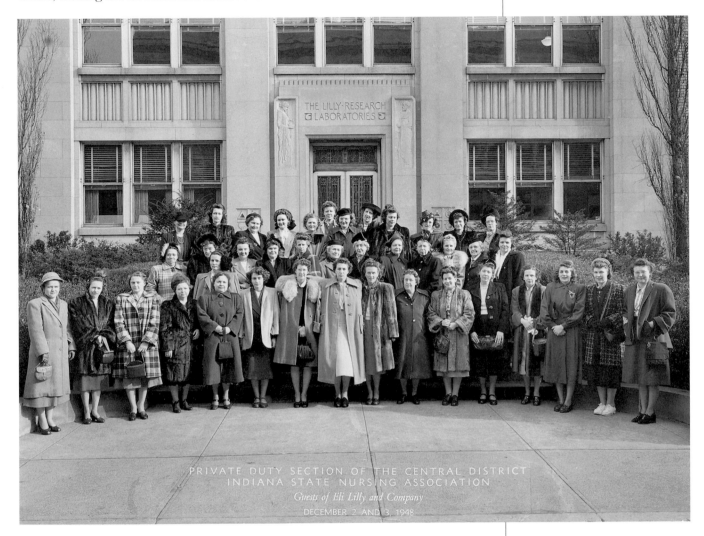

PRIVATE DUTY SECTION OF THE CENTRAL DISTRICT
INDIANA STATE NURSING ASSOCIATION
Guests of Eli Lilly and Company
DECEMBER 2 AND 3, 1948

The Private Duty Section of ISNA's Central District in December 1948 visited Eli Lilly and Company's laboratory in Indianapolis. (ISNA Collection M0380, Indiana Historical Society)

The ISNA's efforts to help keep its members up to date continued. The *AJN* Committee helped "the association have a better informed membership by stimulating among its members a greater use of information, news, articles, and services" provided in the professional magazine. *AJN* subscriptions rose from 178 in 1939 to 397 in 1940, due in large part to personal contacts made by committee and district members.[34] In 1951 ISNA's magazine, the *Lamp*, first published in 1937, officially changed its name to the *Indiana Nurse*.

Executive Secretary Helen Teal retired on 1 May 1947. At the convention that year, members held a banquet for her, where her colleague, Mary Maloney, executive secretary of the West Virginia State Nurses Association, recalled Miss Teal's commitment to the ISNA:

I want to tell the home folks gathered here a little about the convention habits of this Teal they sponsored....She is one of those front seat get there early delegates who pricks up her ears like a thoroughbred: thinks deeply, understands quickly, and challenges the speakers sometimes in a very convincing way, with this State of Indiana and you, as her constituents in her mind. I'm sure she always brings home the bacon. The progress in this state exemplifies this fact.[35]

Helen Teal was unique in the ISNA history for serving as its first full-time executive secretary.

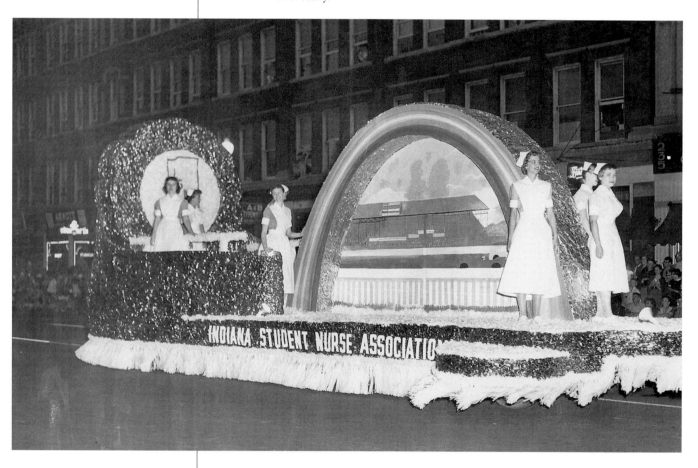

Indiana Student Nurses Association float in the 1957 Indianapolis 500 Parade (ISNA Collection M0380, Indiana Historical Society)

Organizational changes reflected the ISNA's growth. In the 1940s there were three nursing sections: Private Duty, Public Health, and Industrial Nursing. To deal with nurses' employment problems in hospitals, the association established the Institutional Nursing section in 1947. This split into two divisions in 1948 with the introduction of the Administrators and General Duty sections. The cramped space in the ISNA headquarters led to the creation of a Housing Committee in 1950 and a move to larger quarters in the "Terminal

Building" in April 1951. Also in 1951 the first meeting of the Indiana State Student Nurses Association was held. The first meeting of the Executive Committee on Educational Administrators, Consultants, and Teachers was held in 1953.[36] Then in 1954 office nurses met for the first time as a conference group of the Special Group section.

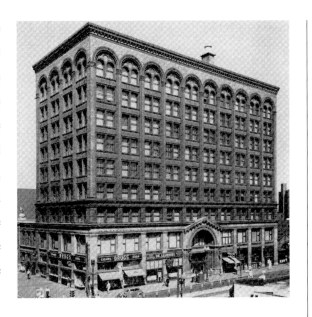

ISNA moved its offices from the Circle Tower to the Terminal Building in April 1951. According to printed reports, the "move to larger quarters was urgently needed." (ISNA Archives, *The Indiana Nurse*, April 1951, page 7)

"The Army Needs Nurses!" (Once Again)

War broke out in Korea in June 1950, and the ISNA again responded. In April 1951 the *Indiana Nurse* announced, "The Army Needs Nurses!", and it emphasized that only two of Indiana's quota of fifty-two had reported for duty. The ad also called for schools of nursing to help stimulate interest in Army nursing, and it reported that a new film, *Army Nurse Corps Begins 50th Year*, was available for viewing by nursing students.[37] During the three years of conflict, only 500 of the 5,500 members of the Army Nurse Corps received assignments in Korea. In addition, three hospital ships rotated as station hospitals in Korean waters. On one of these, the USS *Repose*, was Lieutenant Adelaide Wilhemon from Indiana. As a member of the Navy Nurse Corps, she served ten months aboard the hospital ship and seven months in Korea. The new Department of the Air Force also furnished nurses in the air evacuation of patients.[38]

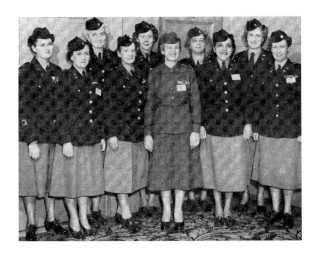

Army nurses attended the 1951 ISNA Annual Meeting. The person in the center of the picture appeared in the new Army Nurse Corps uniform, which was authorized for wear beginning in March 1951. (ISNA Archives, *The Indiana Nurse*, April 1951, page 7)

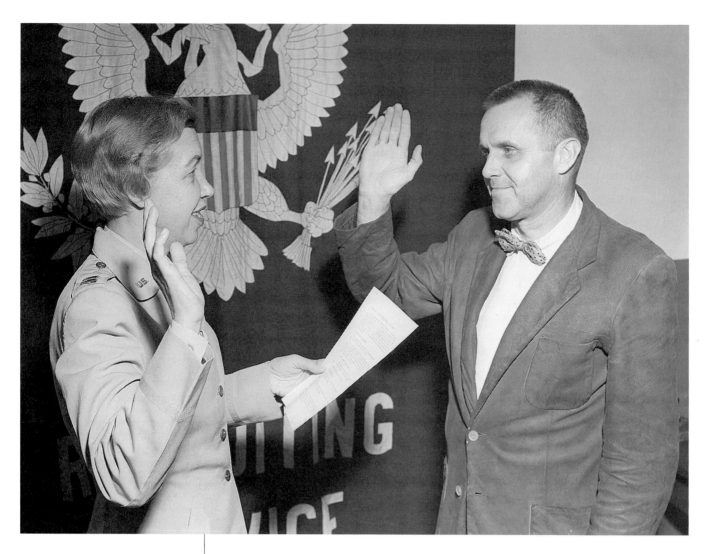

In September 1957 Captain Alma Birath, Army nurse counselor of Indiana, swore in Major Edward Davis (from Madison, Indiana) as the first male nurse to be offered a major commission in the United States Army. The ceremony took place at the recruiting station in Indianapolis. (ISNA Collection M0380, Indiana Historical Society)

Nursing around the Clock: Development of Personnel Policies

At the first annual convention since the end of the war, the main discussions focused on establishing standardized personnel policies. In 1947 Mary York, chair of the newly formed Institution section, became one of the ISNA representatives on the joint committee with the Indiana Hospital Association that addressed issues of long working hours and nurse/patient ratios. At the 1947 section meeting, she reported that hospital nurses were in a crisis and outlined personnel policies "that had to take place immediately." These included reducing the nurse/patient ratio, clarifying withholding taxes, allowing nurses to live away from the hospital, developing standard routines, establishing minimum salary rates, changing work hours to forty-four hours per week initially and eventually moving to a forty-hour workweek, adding one day of sick leave a month, adding two weeks of vacation time and progressing to three, and developing a differential salary rate for 3–11 and 11–7 shifts.[39]

Personnel policy reform was an issue for several years to come. At the 1948 convention, the results of the joint study by the ISNA and the Indiana Hospital Association were reported. Based on a review of fifty hospitals' personnel policies, the survey showed that nurses were working six to seven days a week with two weeks of vacation and one month of sick time per year.[40] Although nursing associations had begun advocating for an eight-hour day in the 1930s, at the 1953 convention the House of Delegates adopted a resolution to support a forty-hour, five-day workweek for nurses. That same year, Indianapolis City Hospital (renamed Marion County General Hospital) implemented a forty-hour workweek. By 1957 the hospital was promising graduate nurse recruits not only a forty-hour week but also premiums for evening and night shifts, compensation for overtime, three weeks vacation, accumulation of thirty-six days of sick leave, and participation in employee hospitalization plans. Other changes were in motion as well. By the mid-1950s black nursing students at Marion County General Hospital were no longer segregated in their own quarters and were included in planned social activities.[41]

Student nurses from Indianapolis General Hospital go caroling in the 1950s. (From the collection of the Wishard Nursing Museum)

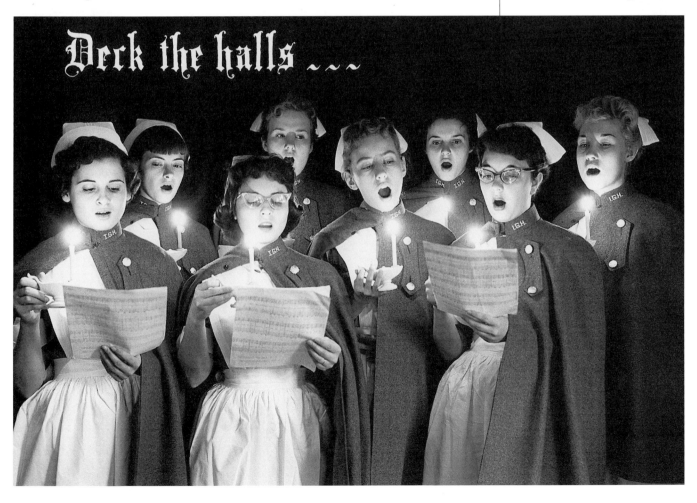

"To Dwell Together in Unity": Inter-Group Relations

In 1948 seven southern states and the District of Columbia still barred African American nurses from membership in their state associations. At that time the ANA offered them individual membership. In the other states, including Indiana, African American nurses could join the ANA through the regular channels of district and state associations. Then in 1950 the ANA House of Delegates ushered in a policy of full participation of minority groups in the asso-

The ISNA Inter-Group Relations meeting in 1957. Pictured (top to bottom) are: Genevieve Beghtel, ISNA president; Mildred Adams, chairman, Inter-Group Relations program committee; Florence Brown, ISNA assistant executive secretary; Margaret Hawkins, committee member who presided at one of the meetings. Also pictured is Grace Maar, wearing the corsage, from the American Nurses Association's Inter-Group Relations Department. (ISNA Collection M0380, Indiana Historical Society)

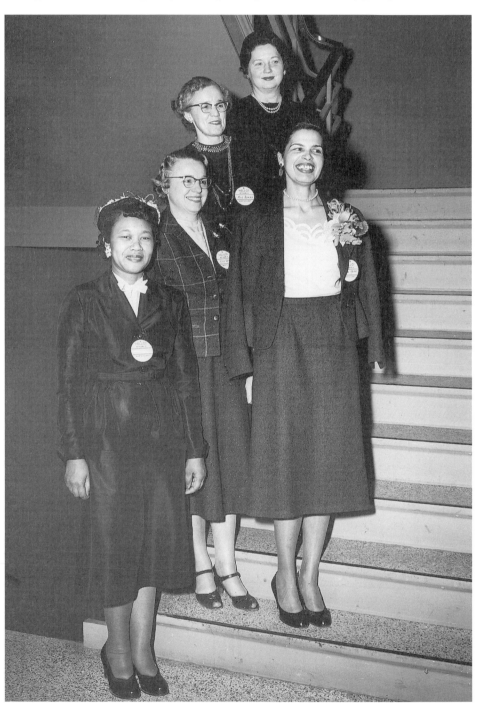

ciation. A year later, the National Association of Colored Graduate Nurses (NACGN), which had formed in 1908, dissolved. Hailing this momentous move, Mabel Staupers, the NACGN's president, stated:

> *Neither health nor disease know man-made barriers….United in a common cause for the benefit of humanity, all nurses can work together, sharing opportunities as well as responsibilities, to the end that this world of ours may become increasingly better.*[42]

Following the ANA's lead, in 1952 the ISNA formed the Inter-Group Relations Committee to remove any barriers to membership. This committee brought recommendations to the ISNA House of Delegates following a survey of the state's nursing schools. A 1954 survey showed 79 percent of schools in Indiana enrolled students regardless of race. That same year, in *Brown v. Board of Education*, the Supreme Court unanimously overturned the "separate but equal" doctrine, thereby outlawing segregation. At the 1956 Annual Convention, the Inter-Group Relations Committee reported that 100 percent of all Indiana nursing schools enrolled students regardless of their race.[43]

Also in the 1950s the *Indiana Nurse* began showing greater diversity in its articles. For example, in 1951 it featured Elizabeth Fisher Scott from the Division of School Health, Health and Hospital Corporation of Marion County, who worked as a public health nurse on a Navajo Indian Reservation.[44] Then in 1957 it highlighted the ISNA's first Inter-Group Relations Institute held in Indianapolis in February. Significantly, the journal emphasized:

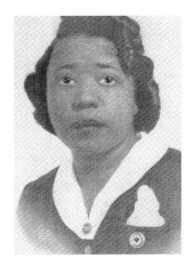

Elizabeth Fisher Scott was a staff nurse with the Division of School Health, Health and Hospital Corporation during the 1950s in Indianapolis. She spent time working with the Navajo in Arizona and wrote about her experiences in *The Indiana Nurse*. (ISNA Archives, *The Indiana Nurse*, February 1956, page 7)

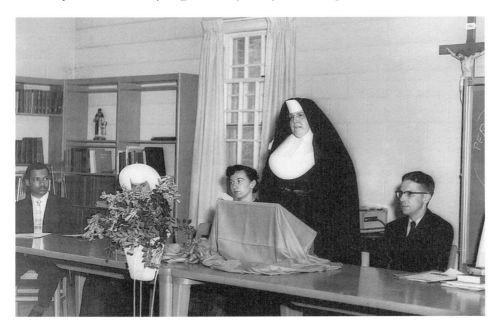

A 1957 mental health discussion at the Holy Cross School of Nursing in South Bend. Indicative of the time, there was this hand-written note on the back of the photograph: "Kindly do not crop panelist at left. We are proud of our interracial group." (ISNA Collection M0380, Indiana Historical Society)

America is a nation of minority groups—racial, religious and national and all of us, regardless of our background, at times have found ourselves in the difficult position of being in the minority group—and with the feeling of being alone and misunderstood....Each of us needs to inform himself for so often we are isolated from, or unaware of, the problems of the society around us.[45]

In 1957 Robert Gordon, Indiana regional director of the Anti-Defamation League of B'nai B'rith, eloquently spoke at the ISNA annual convention about race relations. His presentation, "To Dwell Together in Unity," spoke of humankind's struggles with race issues and expressed the hope for change that was now possible:

Private organizations, such as your own professional agency, have performed wonders in analyzing the problem of prejudice and discrimination and suggesting workable and valid solutions to the problems. More and more bigoted behavior is becoming branded with anti-social stigma and society is beginning to isolate those who seek to poison the human mind with the deadly germs of hate.[46]

ISNA representatives to the 1958 American Nurses Association convention in Atlantic City, New Jersey. (L to R) Mary Ann Robertson, Kathryn Lawson, Jane Lee Jenkins, Thelma Sanders, Norma Mattingly, Louise Phillabaum, Norma Jean Watkins, Pearl Long, and Wilma Green. (ISNA Collection M0380, Indiana Historical Society)

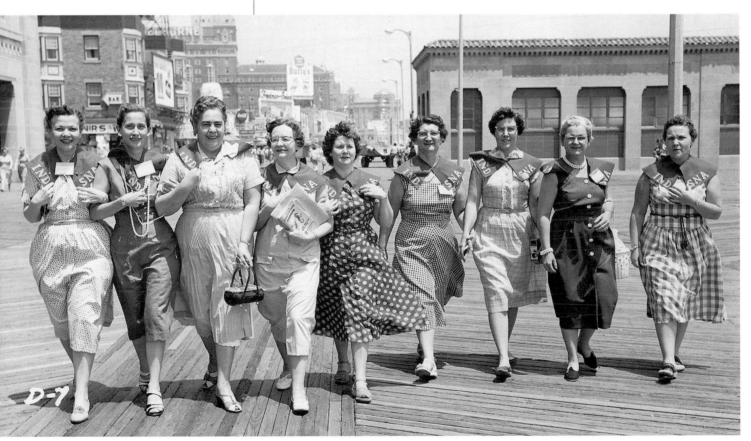

ISNA Golden Anniversary

At the 1953 Annual Convention, President Helen Weber summed up the association's first fifty years as "50 Years of Accomplishments and 50 Years of Surmounted Difficulties." Part of the celebration consisted of recognizing senior nurses who had been active in professional nursing for forty years or more. A highlight of the three-day convention was a historical skit of the ISNA's development, presented by nursing students from Fort Wayne Lutheran, St. Joseph, and Methodist Hospitals. Then at the closing banquet, Archbishop John Francis Noll paid tribute to thirteen Indiana nurses who gave their lives during World War II.[47]

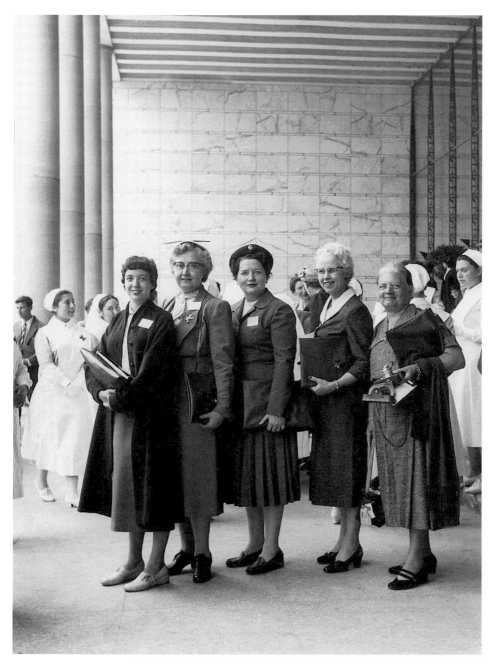

Pictured at left are five of the twelve Indiana nurses who attended the 11th Quadrennial Congress of the International Council of Nurses paused outside the Congress headquarters in Rome in May 1957.
(L to R) Suzanne Jackson, student nurse; Elsie Norman; Genevieve Beghtel; Martha Warstler; and Inez Stierwalt.
(ISNA Collection M0380, Indiana Historical Society)

ISNA members continued to derive great satisfaction from service to their country, their members, and their patients. Using traditional feminine ideals, President Helen Weber concluded her 1953 Presidential Address by stating, "Above all things, we have a right to win personal and professional happiness. Happiness is won through loving service—not by being loved, but by giving love."[48] As the 1950s came to a close, however, this rhetoric would change to reflect the social unrest of the 1960s. The theme of the 1959 Annual Convention reflected the sign of the times: "Nursing in the Atomic Age."[49] By then, the ISNA membership was at an all-time high of 4,489 nurses in eighteen districts.[50]

———•◆•———

Endnotes

[1]Susan Shoemaker, "Opening remarks," 1940 ISNA Annual Convention, Box 5, folder 1, IHS.

[2]Sister Theresa, Invocation, 1940 ISNA Convention.

[3]President's Address, 1941 ISNA Annual Convention, Box 5, folder 3, IHS.

[4]Annual Report, Box 5, folder 1, 1940, IHS.

[5]Mary M. Schroder, "History of the Indiana State Nurses' Association" (M.A. thesis, University of Chicago, 1958), Box 13, folder 1, 1958, IHS.

[6]Nursing Council for War Services—Correspondence and Papers, 1941–1945, Box 25, folder 9, IHS.

[7]Nursing Council.

[8]Annual Report, 1942 ISNA Annual Convention, Box 5, folder 5, IHS.

[9]President's Address, 1942 ISNA Convention.

[10]Hester Anne Hale, *Caring for the Community: The History of Wishard Hospital* (Indianapolis: Wishard Memorial Foundation, 1999), 83.

[11]Annual Report, 1943 ISNA Annual Convention, Box 5, folder 7, IHS.

[12]1943 Annual Report.

[13]Annual Report of the Educational Director, 1940, Box 5, folder 2.

[14]Annual Report, 1940, Box 5, folder 2, IHS.

[15]1942 Annual Report.

[16]Press Release, 1942 ISNA Annual Convention, Box 5, folder 6, IHS.

[17]1946 Annual Report.

[18]Annual Report, 1947 ISNA Annual Convention, Box 5, folder 12, IHS.

[19]Annual Report, 1953 ISNA Annual Convention, Box 7, folder 1, IHS.

[20]Julia Kirk Blackwelder, *Now Hiring: The Feminization of Work in the United States, 1900–1995* (College Station, Texas A&M University Press, 1997), 151–154.

[21]Philip Kalisch and Beatrice Kalisch, *The Advance of American Nursing*, 3rd ed. (Philadelphia: J. B. Lippincott Co., 1995), 372.

[22]Presidential Address, 1947, Box 5, folder 11, IHS.

[23]"Report of the Indiana State Board of Examination and Registration of Nurses and the ISNA," Box 5, folder 12, IHS.

[24]1947 Annual Report, Private Duty Section, Box 5, folder 12, IHS.

[25]Presidential Address, 5 March 1948, Box 6, folder 2, IHS.

[26]1948 ISNA Annual Convention, Box 6, folder 3, IHS.

[27]Ibid.

[28]Barbara Melosh, *"The Physician's Hand": Work Culture and Conflict in American Nursing* (Philadelphia: Temple University Press, 1982), 46–47, 182.

[29] *The Indiana Nurse*, April 1952.

[30] Marjorie Lentz Porter, "A Case Study of the Organizational Lifecycle of the DePauw University School of Nursing, 1954–1994" (Ed.D. diss., Indiana University, 2001); Dotaline E. Allen, *History of Nursing in Indiana* (Indianapolis: Wolfe Publishing Co., 1950), 82; Helen R. Johnson, "History of Purdue University's Nursing Education Programs" (Ed.D. diss., Indiana University, 1975); Deborah A. Barnhart, ed., *Caring for the Past and Future: An Historical Perspective, 1963–1988* (Terre Haute: Indiana State University School of Nursing, 1988).

[31] Presidential Address, Box 5, folder 11, IHS.

[32] Advisory Council Minutes, Box 7, folder 3, IHS.

[33] Box 5 folder 7, 1943; Schroder, "History," 29–30, IHS.

[34] 1940 Annual Report.

[35] 1947 Tribute Banquet Presentation, Box 5, folder 12, IHS.

[36] Annual Meetings, Box 7, folder 2, IHS.

[37] "The Army Needs Nurses," *The Indiana Nurse* (April 1951): 6.

[38] Kalisch and Kalisch, 381–382; and "News About Nurses," *The Indiana Nurse* (April 1952): 17.

[39] 1947 ISNA Annual Convention, Box 5, folder 12, IHS.

[40] 1948 ISNA Annual Convention, Box 6, folder 4, IHS.

[41] Hale, 97–99.

[42] Mabel K. Staupers, "Story of the National Association of Colored Graduate Nurses," *AJN* 51, no. 4 (April 1951): 223.

[43] 1956 Annual Report, IHS.

[44] Elizabeth Fisher Scott, "Public Health Nursing—On the Navajo," *The Indiana Nurse* (1956): 7–8.

[45] "Institute Considers Minority Problems," *The Indiana Nurse* (1957): 4–5.

[46] Robert Gordon, Presentation at ISNA Convention, 19 October 1957, Box 8, folder 1, IHS.

[47] 1953 ISNA Annual Convention, Box 7, folder 2, IHS.

[48] Ibid.

[49] Suzanne Parr and Toby Etchels, "Serving the Profession Since 1903," *The Indiana Nurse* (1993): 63–69.

[50] Schroder, 73.

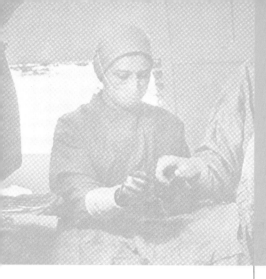

Chapter 5

"The Times They Are A-Changin'"
1960-1980

Linda Rodebaugh, Ed.D., R.N.

Civil Defense nurses participated in a mock disaster drill in 1960. Mary Spangler (foreground) and Vera May Maynard assist Dr. J. F. Hinchman in caring for "casualties." (ISNA Collection M0380, Indiana Historical Society)

Bob Dylan's album *The Times They Are A-Changin'* was released in January 1964 and said much about the decades of the 1960s and 1970s. Nationwide, general unrest was evident in response to the nuclear threat associated with the Cold War and the Cuban Missile Crisis. In addition, the Civil Rights movement and the Vietnam conflict contributed to youth unrest on college campuses across the country. It was the time of the Great Society and the Medicare bill. As the

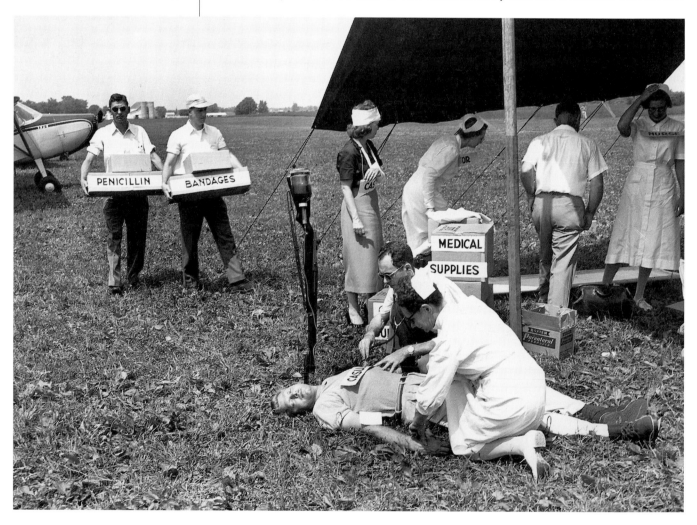

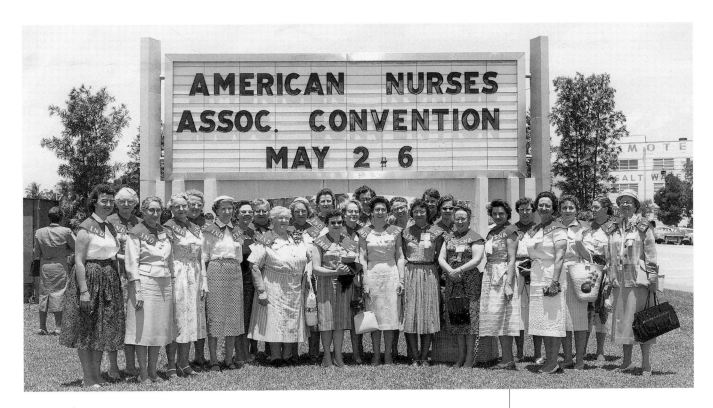

1970s dawned, health care was the third largest industry in the United States, and rapidly increasing hospital costs became a concern of the public and the federal government.[1]

Many of these social issues were of concern to nurses involved in the ISNA as reflected in both district and state program planning. Programs about drug abuse appeared, and nurses learned about responding to disaster, thereby making civil defense programs plentiful. In May 1960 the ANA convention featured the film "Civil Defense, Emergency Hospital" produced by the Federal Civil Defense Administration. The following month, the *Indiana Nurse* headlined: "Mr. C. D. Is Pleased to Announce a One-Day Institute on Saturday, June 11, 1960."[2] To provide up-to-date information on civil defense, the program included information regarding the sorting of casualties and the organization and functions of the County Civil Defense Medical Services Committee. Other ISNA programs focused on radioactive fallout and bomb shelters, water and food needs, sanitation guidelines, and basic first aid information.[3]

As is often the case, interest peaked in disaster preparedness following a crisis. In this case, the numerous tornadoes across Indiana on Palm Sunday, April 1965, sparked action. Statewide, the devastation was massive in property loss and especially in the number of lives lost. As noted in the 1965 Annual Report from District 12:

Delegates to the 1960 American Nurses Association convention in Miami posed for a photo outside their hotel. (ISNA Collection M0380, Indiana Historical Society)

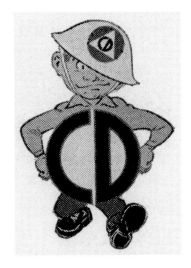

Mr. CD Man was depicted in advertisements for civil defense in the *Indiana Nurse*. (ISNA Archives)

Many of us realized, perhaps for the first time how essential it is that we as professionally trained persons give some thought to being prepared to serve in this capacity. We can agree more than ever before with the statement made by the ANA Special Committee on Disaster Preparedness... "Nurses must develop the attitude that in all disasters they must be able to do the best for the most with the least by the fewest."[4]

"Difficult, Possibly Hazardous, Working Conditions"

As the United States's involvement in Vietnam expanded, the Army Nurse Corps called for 500 nurses who would serve as commissioned officers. American nurses first went to Vietnam in 1962, but after the war escalated in 1965, the plea for nurses became much louder. Once again, the ISNA assisted in nurse recruitment. In 1965 the *Indiana Nurse* announced, "As the number of casualties grow, so grows the need for medical care—the best medical care that our Nation can provide for those who serve her." Drawing on patriotic rhetoric mixed with an enticing sense of adventure, it continued, "Excellent opportunities await the registered nurse for commissioned service in modern facilities all over the world, plus the satisfaction of knowing you are doing your part in the defense of your country and the Free World."[5] Qualified nurses could request a guaranteed assignment to one of eleven Army hospitals stateside, or selected overseas areas in Okinawa, Korea, or Germany. Nurse anesthetists and operating room nurses could request a guaranteed assignment to Vietnam.

Then in 1966 the *Indiana Nurse* advertised for civilian nurses to go to Vietnam:

This ad appeared in the December 1966 edition of the *Indiana Nurse*. Thousands of registered nurses were needed during the Vietnam War. The ad promises "difficult, possibly hazardous, working conditions...in remote locations." (ISNA Archives)

CIVILIAN REGISTERED NURSES

NEEDED IN

VIET NAM

AGENCY FOR INTERNATIONAL DEVELOPMENT
U.S. DEPARTMENT OF STATE

Difficult, possibly hazardous, working conditions; long hours, great responsibility, in remote locations. To work with international medical teams in provincial hospitals of South Viet Nam, treating civilian war casualties and villagers needing medical attention, as part of U.S. AID program.

Applicants must be U.S. citizens for at least 5 years, without dependents, physically fit, and willing to serve abroad for at least 18 months.

Requires Registered Nurse Certificate and at least 2 years ward nursing experience.

Salary range: $6,500-$10,000, plus 25% hardship bonus, housing allowance, and other benefits.

TO APPLY

Interviews will be held January 16 through 21 from 11:00 a.m. to 7:00 p.m. at 623 South Wabash Avenue, Chicago, Illinois 60605. For information or appointments call Area Code 312 353-6530 (call collect if out of town). After January 21 information may be obtained by writing the Far East Recruitment Division, Agency for International Development, Washington, D.C.

A.I.D. is an Equal Opportunity Employer

DECEMBER, 1966   9

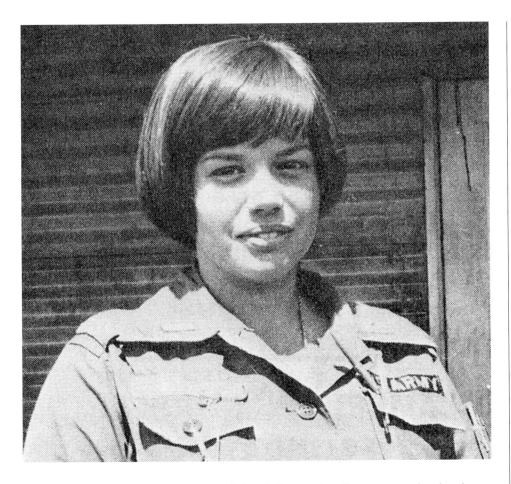

Army 1st Lt. Mary Heath from Indianapolis served in Vietnam with the 18th Surgical Hospital. (ISNA Archives, *The Indiana Nurse*, March 1967, page 21)

Second Lieutenant Karren E. Mundell was the first woman in the Army Nurse Corps from Indiana to volunteer for direct assignment in Vietnam. She served for one year during 1966–1967. Prior to entering the Army in April 1966, the 1965 graduate of Indiana University worked in labor and delivery at the Coleman Hospital for Women in Indianapolis. While in Vietnam, she was a general-duty staff nurse in the intensive care recovery ward at the First Logistical Command's Third Surgical Hospital, located at the Bien Hoa Air Base. The hospital was a compact sixty-bed facility, specifically designed and equipped for the treatment of battle casualties. [6]

Wartime nursing could have certain advantages. *The Indiana Nurse* quoted Second Lieutenant Mundell: "I'm really impressed with the opportunities offered by the Army. The pay is equal to or better than in civilian hospitals. Also, I've had a chance to visit several areas of Vietnam, and have been to Bangkok, Thailand. Before I leave this country, I also plan to spend a few days in Hong Kong." [7]

Mostly, however, wartime nursing was "difficult" and "hazardous," as the ad intimated. Nurses who served in Vietnam were close to the fighting front. With the arrival of *Dustoff*, the helicopter chopper ambulance, a wounded soldier could be in surgery within twenty minutes of being injured. With the combination of helicopter evacuation and skilled surgical teams, mortality rates decreased from as high as 7 percent during World War II to 1 percent in Vietnam.[8] Soon after her arrival in Vietnam in June 1966, Second Lieutenant Mundell wrote:

> *We had a couple of "dust-offs" last night and I went over to pre-op to help. The ones you can help make you feel so good but the ones we can't tear me apart inside. They're all so young. The young fellow we gave 97 units of blood to last week died on my shift. It's almost more than a person can stand and the doctor who's been here a year assured me that I would never get use[d] to it. I imagine he's right.*[9]

In February 1967 she wrote in cryptic description of the unspeakable horror of war: "We've had another real bad patient. I specialed him yesterday. He's on a respirator—a leg gone—very bad." Near the end of her tour of duty, she had

Military news was a regular feature in the *Indiana Nurse* during the Vietnam War. This photo appeared in the February 1964 edition. (ISNA Archives)

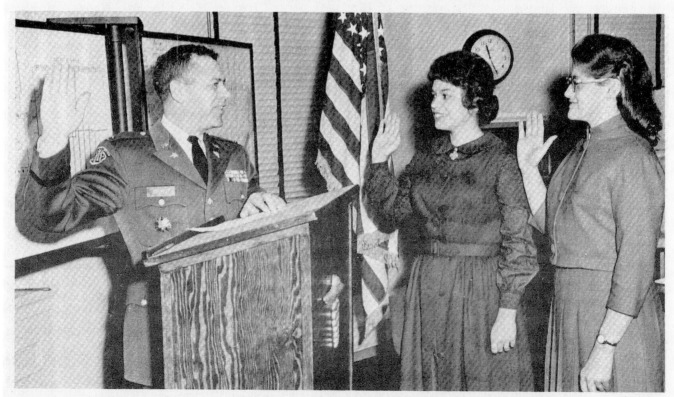

MILITARY NEWS
FATHER COMMISSIONS DAUGHTER AS NURSE

Left to right: Colonel Darrell H. Burnett, Miss Mary Lee Burnett and Miss Ruth E. Roose

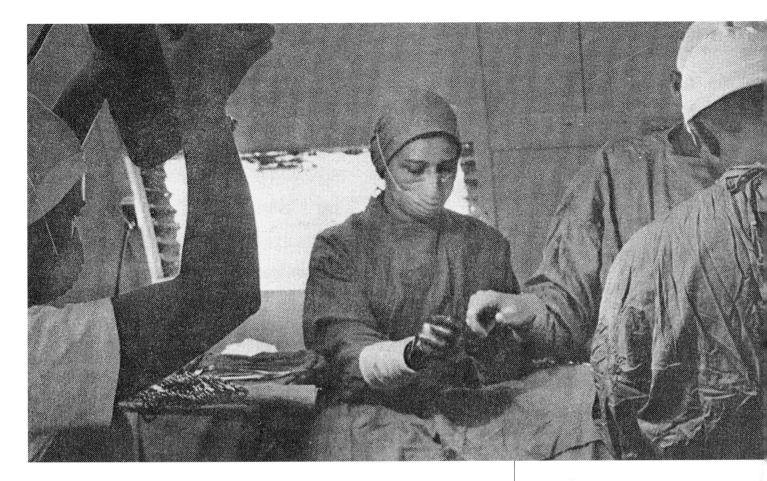

a close call. She wrote home "to reassure you that I'm alive—I'm sure the fact that the V.C. [Viet Cong] mortared the Air Base is in all the news—the mortars landed a good 2 miles away. No problem—Just didn't want you to worry."[10] While Karren Mundell survived her tour, official records indicate eight women nurses and two men nurses from across the United States died from illness or injuries sustained in the Vietnam conflict.

Army nurse 1st Lt. Mary Ann Lemieux (left) from Terre Haute assisted in surgery on a battle-field casualty at the 1st Logistical Command's 7th Surgical Hospital in Cu Chi, Vietnam. In 1967 air-conditioned operating suites and wards were common in all Army hospitals in Vietnam. (ISNA Archives, *The Indiana Nurse*, June 1967, page 21)

Men in White

In 1960 men continued to constitute the smallest nursing minority, accounting for only 1 percent of the 440,000 active nurses.[11] In 1964 of the twenty-four schools of nursing (baccalaureate, associate, and diploma programs) accredited by the Indiana State Board of Nurses' Registration and Nursing Education, eleven continued to refuse admission to males. Of the ten accredited practical schools in Indiana, half did not admit men.[12]

Some strides were made in Indiana around this time, however. At the 62nd Annual ISNA Convention in 1966, Richard O. Hakes of Fort Wayne was elected as the first male president and continued in this position through 1969.[13]

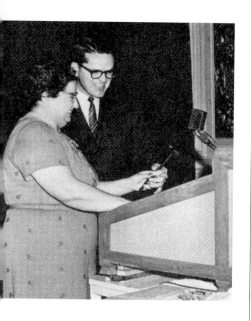

In 1966 Richard O. Hakes of Fort Wayne was the first male to be elected ISNA president. At the organization's annual meeting he was presented with a gavel from outgoing President Marie Loftus. (ISNA Archives, *The Indiana Nurse*, December 1966, page 3)

In December 1970 a faculty member from Holy Cross School of Nursing in South Bend expounded upon the problem of male students' need for clinical experiences in maternity nursing. Faculty "anticipated difficulties in regard to embarrassment for both the student and for the patients receiving maternity nursing care."[14] While the patient was their primary concern, faculty also did not want to place the male student in a legally vulnerable situation. Thus, a policy was developed, in cooperation with physicians, which limited the procedures men could perform on women without a female staff member present. Faculty found that "...without exception, patients voiced their acceptance of him as a nurse without regard for his sex. Husbands voiced their relief and encouragement upon seeing a man, like themselves, able to provide support to women in labor and to care for infants competently."[15]

"The Times They Are A-Changin'...Gradually"

Growing pains for the nursing profession continued as nursing care became more technologically complex. Nurses increasingly worked in specialized areas such as cardiac care, which greatly increased their autonomy. This led to tensions among nurses and physicians over what was considered medical practice versus nursing practice. The ISNA frequently received questions regarding what the nurse could legally and ethically do in certain situations. As a case in point, in 1961 nurses from the ANA Committee on Nursing Practice met with representatives from the National League for Nursing, the national occupational health agencies, and the American Heart Association to view the film *External Cardiac Massage* and discuss its implications for nurses. The American Heart Association issued a statement that nurses should be informed about the procedure so they could assist the physician, but that "the procedure itself is a medical one requiring medical diagnosis and should be *initiated only by a physician*." (italics added for emphasis.)[16] The ANA concurred with this belief. Its definition of nursing practice "excludes diagnosis of this nature from the practice of nursing."[17]

In July 1962 the ISNA Committee on Professional Nursing Practice sent questionnaires to directors of hospital nursing services, public health nursing, and all accredited schools of nursing to determine which areas of practice were of most concern to nurses. In particular, apprehension involved intravenous (IV) and venipuncture techniques. Additionally, many voiced concerns over the removal of sutures and packing, performing cardiac massage, pronouncing death, and administering first aid in the emergency room without standing orders. Obstetrical nurses had their own list of concerns that included administering anesthesia in labor and performing rectal exams, sterile vaginal exams, and newborn resuscitation.

In the mid-1960s, the ISNA House of Delegates and the Indiana Hospital Association passed a resolution stating that if nurses were to be expected to start IVs, they must be instructed in the procedure first. The state medical association did not favor the resolution, however, on the grounds that IV therapy was medical practice. As a result, the Indiana State Board of Nursing did not encourage schools to incorporate the teaching of IV therapy.

In 1965 Lucille Wall, executive director of ISNA from 1960 to 1970, clarified the ISNA's stance that "no nurse should be carrying out a practice which she has not been prepared or taught to do."[18] Furthermore, it would be the responsibility of the hospital or agency to provide instruction for the nurse if it expected the nurse to perform such procedures. This was felt to be adequate regarding IV therapy, as the nurse would be following doctor's orders and not making a diagnosis. Lucille Wall added a cautionary warning based on "[today's] practice of 'suing someone for something.' It seems that the health fields are now feeling the impact of such practice."[19]

Closed-chest cardiac resuscitation, however, was a different matter because of the need for immediate action without a medical diagnosis or doctor's order. By 1965 the American Heart Association had changed its original statement from considering it medical practice to now viewing it as an emergency procedure. In summary, Lucille Wall stressed two factors regarding the legal aspects for nurses: the necessity that institutions and/or agencies have written policies, and the responsibility of every professional nurse for her own actions and judgment. Hence, she recommended that each nurse get liability protection.[20]

Joint meetings between various organizations often were fruitful in negotiating specific roles. The ISNA met with the Indiana Hospital Association in 1965 and discussed establishing guidelines for the development of standing orders for emergency room personnel.[21] That same year, the ISNA and the Indiana State Medical Association set up a Liaison Committee to discuss improving nurse-physician relationships and trends in nursing education and service. Members reached consensus regarding the need for cooperation in patient-centered care, the importance of not placing student nurses in positions of major responsibility, and the need for mandatory licensure for Indiana nurses.[22]

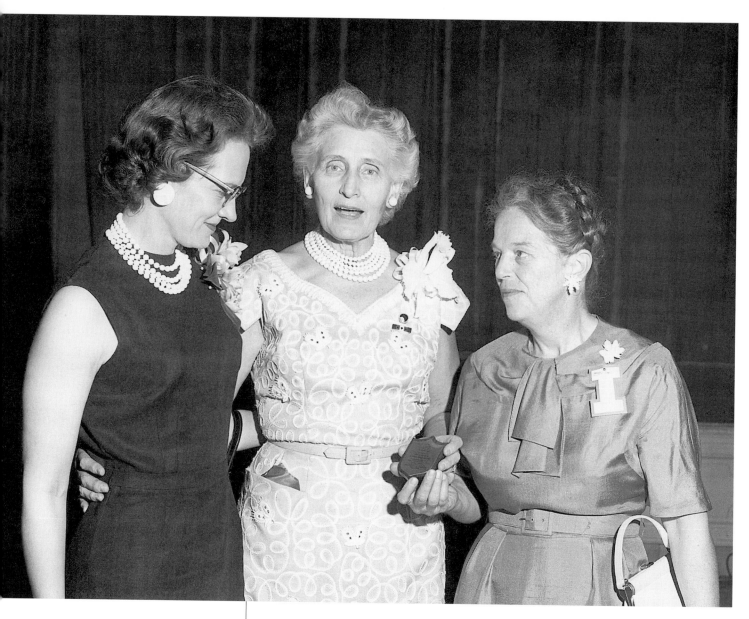

The leadership of the American Nurses Foundation (ANF) in 1962 included (L to R): Georgia Nyland, American Nurses Association third vice president and ANF board member; Katharine Densford Drewes, national campaign chairwoman; and Frances Orgain, ISNA campaign chairwoman. (ISNA Collection M0380, Indiana Historical Society)

Seeds of Unionization

As their work increased in complexity, nurses began agitating for higher salaries. In 1965 the ISNA board approved a beginning annual salary for all staff nurse positions to be $4,500.[23] But any salary increase for nurses lagged behind general increases for other employees nationwide. The Bureau of Labor Statistics for 1963–64 showed that teachers earned on average $6,325; secretaries, $5,170; factory workers, $5,075; and the general-duty nurse in a nonfederal city hospital, $4,500.[24]

In 1967 U.S. Surgeon General William Stewart noted, "[I]ncreases in nurses' salaries will end up in nothing but good."[25] Dr. Stewart spoke favorably of the ANA's goal of a $6,500 annual salary for beginning nurses and also believed it would bring nurses back into the field. Although the AMA supported the salary increase in principle, it questioned the establishment of a minimum rate for the entire country. Rather, each region's supply and demand should determine the nurse's salary.[26]

Many nurses increasingly felt helpless as individuals to improve their economic security and believed their professional associations were not working fast enough to help them. Hence, they began considering unionization and collective bargaining. Some unions had formed in hospitals in the early 1900s, and unionization in general had increased during the Great Depression. In 1937 the ANA board voted against unionization on the grounds that it negated the organization's professional status. Instead, it encouraged members to use their professional organizations to help improve their work situations. Yet, graduate nurses continued to join unions, and in 1943 the California State Nurses Association was the first to agree to be the bargaining representative for its nurses in employment matters. Influenced by this move, in 1946 the ANA officially approved the state nurses associations as collective bargaining agents in all areas affecting nurses' economic security and working conditions.[27]

By the 1960s various hospital administrators tried to assert that the ANA was not really a professional organization but rather a union, which the ANA promptly refuted. It explained the difference in an official statement: "[Whereas] if ANA did not have an economic security program, the association would still exist. If a labor union ceased representing its members, it would no longer have a reason to exist." To allay administrators' anxieties the ANA emphasized: "Where nurses have negotiated matters of working conditions and salary, the collective bargaining technique has proved orderly and effective" and ultimately improved employer-employee relationships and, consequently, patient care.[28]

This ISNA map depicts the twenty-one districts in Indiana. (ISNA Archives)

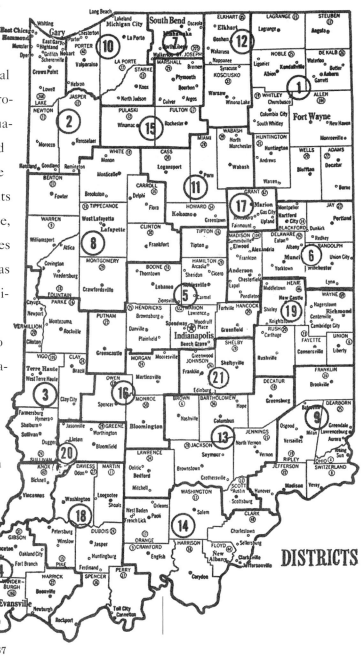

INDIANA STATE NURSES' ASSOCIATION, INC.

DISTRICTS

APRIL, 1967

91

While Indiana did not follow California's lead in assuming a collective bargaining role, the ISNA recognized that the economic and general welfare of nurses influenced the quality and quantity of nursing service. In 1966 the ISNA House of Delegates implemented an active Economic and General Welfare Program tailored to the needs of Indiana nurses. ISNA President Richard Hakes called it one of the most urgent issues facing the ISNA.[29] It adopted several policies, guided by the Minimum Employment Standards for Professional Registered Nurses in Indiana. The ISNA would assist nurses to achieve desired employment standards and help them to avoid employment crises. In conducting its Economic and General Welfare Program, the ISNA would continue to uphold the No-Strike policy adopted by the 1954 House of Delegates.[30]

Entry Level into Practice and Other Educational Issues

In October 1960 the *AJN* celebrated its sixtieth anniversary. To commemorate the event, it included a special supplement titled *Nursing Education—Today*. This topic was specifically chosen as it was noted to be "one of the most widely discussed and controversial in the profession today."[31]

That same year, the Indiana State Medical Association adopted a resolution to encourage colleges and universities in the state to seriously consider starting schools of nursing. Citing the shortage of registered nurses, the resolution asserted that colleges could more effectively administer certain aspects of nursing education. In 1962 reflecting national trends, Indiana's diploma schools still educated 75 percent of nursing students, while baccalaureate programs accounted for only 20 percent and associate degree programs, 4 percent. Yet, one of the ANA's goals was "to insure that, within the next 20–30 years, the education basic to the practice of nursing at the professional level, for those who enter the profession," would be the baccalaureate degree.[32]

In 1963 the Surgeon General's Consultative Group on Nursing issued its pivotal report, *Toward Quality in Nursing*, which found too few nursing schools at the collegiate level, too little research on advancing nursing practice, and too few capable nursing recruits. It called for federal aid to solve the nursing problem, culminating in the Nurse Training Act of 1964, which provided for federal traineeships, scholarships, and money to construct nursing education facilities.[33]

December 1965 was a landmark date for the ANA with the publication of its "ANA Position Paper on Education for Nursing." Citing the current knowledge explosion, the increasing level of education in the United States, and the health care demands of the public, the following position was adopted:

> *The education for all those who are licensed to practice nursing should take place in institutions of higher education....Minimum preparation for beginning professional nursing practice at the present time should be baccalaureate degree education in nursing.... Minimum preparation for beginning technical nursing practice at the present time should be associate degree education in nursing....Education for assistants in the health service occupations should be short, intensive preservice programs in vocational education institutions rather than on-the-job training programs.*[34]

This led to a schism in nursing education as the trend increasingly moved away from the diploma schools to colleges and universities. The federal government continued its financial assistance through Nursing Education Opportunities grants (1967), the Health Manpower Act (1968), and the Nurse Training Act (1971).[35]

In 1967 *Nurses for Indiana, Present and Future* was published. Conducted by the Indiana Committee on Nursing (ICON), the study came to be known as the ICON Report. This detailed study was jointly sponsored by the ISNA, the Indiana League for Nursing, and the Indiana State Board of Nurses' Registration and Nursing Education.[36] Significantly, the ICON Report recommended a state-level nursing education planning body composed of administrators of schools of nursing and appropriate nursing service representatives. Planning was directed toward expanding nursing enrollments and educational facilities, the number and kind of educational programs, the number and quality of clinical facilities, and the cooperative use of those facilities.[37] The ICON Report found that the state was far short of the national average of nurses per 100,000 population, and especially nurses in leadership positions. Thereafter, schools such as Purdue University expanded their associate degree programs to four-year curriculums leading to a Bachelor of Science degree.[38]

In the 1970s the demand for and cost of health care escalated. Medical science achieved great successes in open heart surgery, renal dialysis, and organ transplantation, and this expanding arena created thousands of new nursing jobs.

Aided by the 1971 Nurse Training Act, the number of active RNs across the nation skyrocketed. Graduations from basic nursing programs grew more rapidly during this decade than at any time since 1873. This period also saw an increase in programs leading to the master's degree, which prepared nurses to work as clinical nurse specialists, nurse practitioners, teachers, and administrators.[39] The growth in nursing numbers, however, still could not keep up with the demand.

Education and the nursing shortage were issues in the forefront for the ISNA over the next several years. The House of Delegates revised its bylaws in 1971 to create a Council on Education, which developed the Task Force on

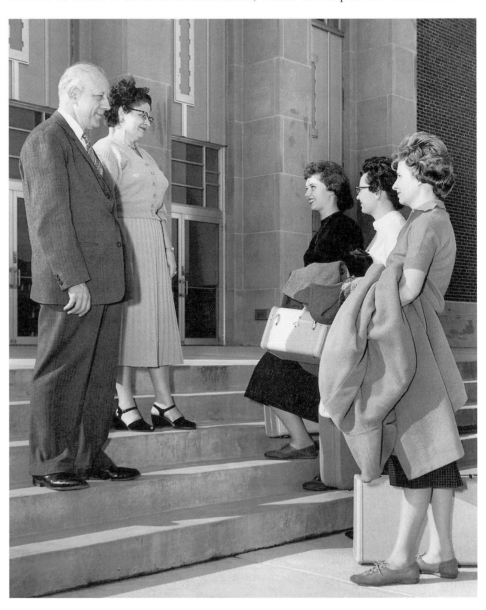

Students are greeted on the steps of Indiana Central College (now University of Indianapolis), which opened an associate degree nursing program in 1959. (ISNA Collection M0380, Indiana Historical Society)

Nursing Needs in Indiana, chaired by Dr. Lois Meier. In 1973 it began developing a statewide plan for nursing education. Deans and directors from all Indiana nursing programs; members of the Council on Education; the Executive Committee of the Conference Group on Nursing Service Administration; staff from Indiana Health Careers Inc.; and members of the State Board of Nurses' Registration and Nursing Education comprised the group. All brought data concerning current enrollments, projected five-year enrollments, program needs and plans for the next two years, and institutional studies of nursing needs in Indiana.[40]

Indiana's Task Force on Nursing Needs concluded that efforts to prepare more nurses for leadership roles in the state were of utmost importance. In 1973 Indiana had three master's degree nursing programs, with two others in the planning phase. There were no doctoral nursing programs, although one was in the early planning stages. The Task Force felt that emphasis for graduate nursing programs should be on the preparation of teachers of nursing, clinical specialists, and nursing service administrators statewide. Additionally, it recommended a graduate program in community health nursing to meet current and projected needs. Indiana University School of Nursing at Indiana University/Purdue University at Indianapolis was given the charge to develop a doctoral program in nursing immediately.[41]

The Task Force indirectly addressed the nursing shortage by recommending that graduate, baccalaureate, associate degree, hospital diploma, and practical nurse programs all continue in order to provide qualified applicants entry into the program of their choice. In the late 1960s and early 1970s, nurse practitioners were in evidence in several parts of the country, and the Indiana Task Force encouraged nursing schools to support the new nurse practitioner programs consistent with emerging national trends. The state master plan also stressed the necessity of continuing education for all nursing levels due to rapidly changing technology. Last, the Task Force concluded that ways to provide greater financial support for nursing programs were needed.[42]

Some improvements in nursing education were made. Diploma schools in the state continued their downward spiral: by 1974, only 28 percent of graduates trained in diploma schools, while the number of associate degree programs rose to 41 percent and baccalaureate programs to 31 percent.[43]

During this time, the ISNA Council on Education continued the discussion about differentiation between the baccalaureate and associate degree nurse and entry level into practice. "Decision Time in '79" was the theme for the 1979 ISNA Biennial Convention, and the topic of entry level into practice promised to be heavily debated. Delegates passed a resolution to make the baccalaureate degree in nursing the minimum educational preparation. Furthermore, it resolved:

That the ISNA Commissions on Education, Nursing Services and Practice develop a timetable for implementation of the resolution in Indiana by 1981 which clearly delineates grandfathering of currently licensed practitioners, competencies, title and projected availability of/and requirement for RN manpower prepared at the BSN level for the future, and that such a timetable be presented to this House in 1981.[44]

Although the resolution passed, no legislation was ever adopted in Indiana related to entry level into practice.[45]

Continuing Education Begins

With an emphasis on *learning* as opposed to *earning* credits, continuing education programs blossomed as the concept of education as a lifelong practice grew in response to the knowledge explosion of the 1970s.[46] In 1973 Jean E. Schweer; Dr. Mary Anne Roehm; and Geraldine Wojtowicz, with financial support from the U.S. Public Health Service, initiated the Indiana Statewide Continuing Education Planning project. Dr. Charlotte Carlley was the initial project director. Beginning 1 January 1974, through grant monies from the Kellogg Foundation, the Indiana Statewide Program for Continuing Education in Nursing was developed and implemented over a three-year period with Dr. Belinda Puetz as project director. At the close of the grant period, the ISNA assumed the project's activities and Dr. Puetz remained the director. She received additional Kellogg funding to continue the project.[47] In 1979 the ANA accredited the ISNA as a provider and approver of continuing education.

For a period of time during the late 1970s, the ISNA debated continuing-education legislation as a requirement for license renewal. Although ISNA President Kathryn Lawson supported continuing education for nurses, she noted in 1976 that there was "no research available to clearly demonstrate any change or improvement in practice as a result of participation" in it.[48] Along with the entry-into-practice issue, delegates debated the continuing education question at the 1979 ISNA Biennial Convention, but they did not adopt a resolution for mandatory continuing education for license renewal.

The ISNA Comes of Age

As the association grew, the *Indiana Nurse* underwent many changes in format, distribution frequency, and content. Initially published six times a year, it became a quarterly publication in 1962. Financing the magazine was a never-ending concern, and the ISNA board increased its advertising in 1961. Due to problems with implementing this plan, however, only one ad for an item unrelated to nursing or medicine ever appeared. Relying on the female subscription base, the ad titled "The New, Better Duncan Hines Food and Vegetable Cutter" appeared in the March 1961 issue.[49]

Due to financial constraints, in 1975 the ISNA suspended quarterly publication of the *Indiana Nurse* and published only preconvention issues after that time. The first issue of the *ISNA Bulletin* was published in January 1975. Statewide, membership increased as evidenced by the creation of additional districts during those two decades. By 1967 the association had twenty-one districts.

Beginning in the 1960s nursing issues became the focus of unprecedented political activity, and the ANA and state associations became even more active in the public arena. To cover costs, in 1963 the ANA increased dues from $7.50 to $12.50. By 1969 the national association was deeply in debt, however, and it raised dues in 1970. Denoting an increasing sense of urgency in dealing with national health policy,

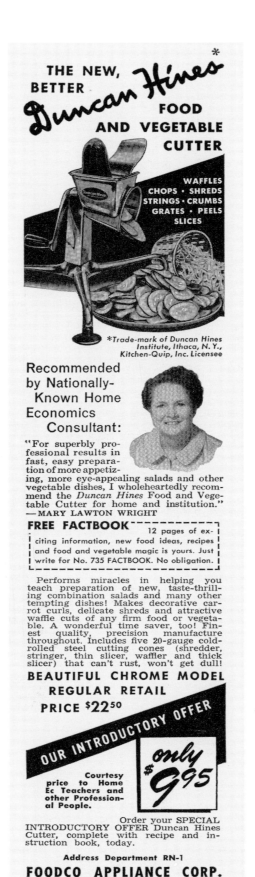

This Duncan Hines food and vegetable cutter was the only nonmedical product ever to be advertised in *The Indiana Nurse*. The fine print indicated the $9.95 introductory offer was a "courtesy price to Home Ec Teachers and other Professional People." (ISNA Archives)

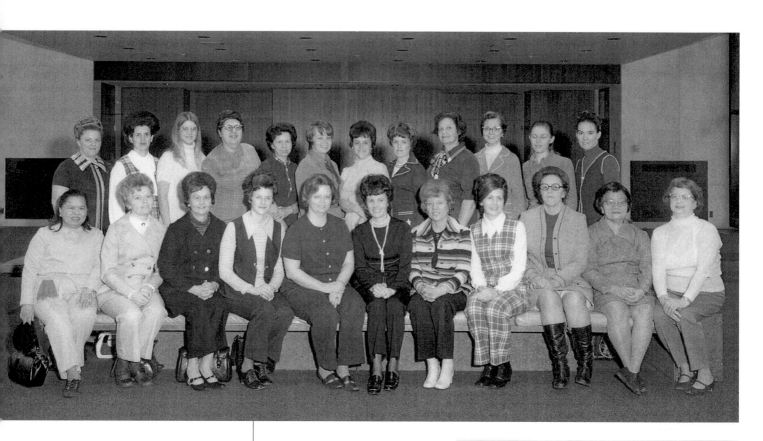

ISNA members from District 18 visited Eli Lilly and Company's world headquarters in Indianapolis on February 7, 1972. (Courtesy of Daviess Community Hospital, Washington, Indiana)

The hard work, dedication, and contribution of nurses were recognized on this U.S. postage stamp in 1960. (ISNA Collection M0380, Indiana Historical Society)

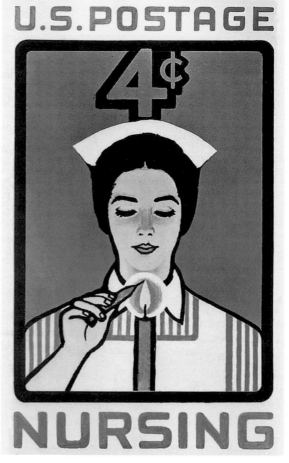

the ANA raised dues yet again in 1976 to total $40. In 1977 annual dues for a member of the ISNA totaled $65, which were paid in addition to and at the same time as the dues for the ANA.[50]

"Behold! The Turtle Moves Only When His Neck Is Out"[51]

Although these words appeared in 1961 from ISNA President Dorothy Damewood, they appropriately described the legislative achievements of the 1970s. The first dealt with the Nurse Practice Act and nursing's scope of practice. Prior to 1971 Indiana nurses were held to the first statutory definition of the practice of nursing that had been passed in 1949. This definition addressed dependent functions only and did not define nursing practice itself, but rather focused on the services for which the registered nurse received compensation.[52] The 1949 definition remained unchanged until 1971 when the first substantive changes finally occurred. This revision focused on identifying more specific nursing practice activities, but because of the manner in which it was written, "everything was interpreted to be as prescribed by a licensed physician....So the scope of registered nursing practice was defined within the dependent context," stated Dr. Brenda Lyon, former ISNA president.[53]

ISNA Board of Directors in 1978 (ISNA Collection M0380, Indiana Historical Society)

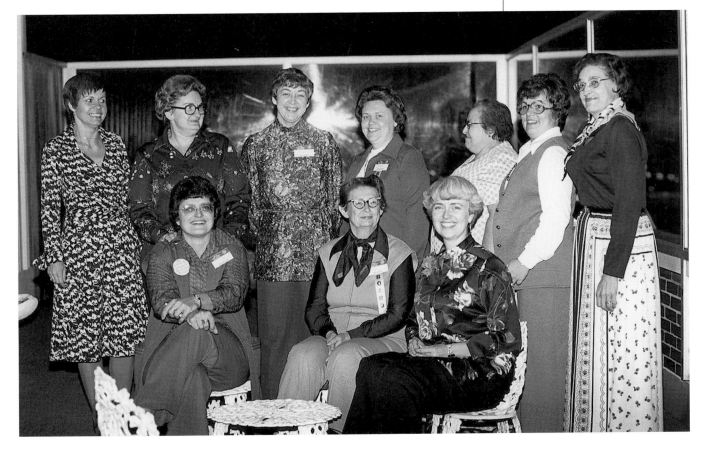

Members of the ISNA Legislative Committee worked with the Indiana House and Senate on revision to the Nurse Practice Act of 1975. Committee members joined Governor Otis Bowen, M.D., as he signed the bill into law. Pictured are (L to R): Lucretia Ann Saunders, ISNA executive director; Norma Wallman; Linda J. Shinn, ISNA associate executive director; Governor Bowen; Brenda Lyon, chair, ISNA Legislative Committee; Jean Grimsley, ISNA president.

The major ISNA endeavor in the early 1970s was to separate out nursing's autonomous scope of practice from the delegated authority scope of practice. The ISNA Legislative Committee worked on a definition of nursing practice from 1971 to 1974. Following historical precedents, they sought support from influential persons and organizations, obtaining feedback from the ISNA members and the Indiana State Medical Association. Two challenges persisted in the process. The first involved physicians from the medical association who took exception to the use of the term "nursing diagnosis." Physicians came around after the nurses encouraged them to look solely at the dictionary definition of the word diagnosis: "conclusion one makes after having collected data." Dr. Lyon described the second challenge: "We were writing a definition to make it clear what nurses were responsible for, what the public should be able to count

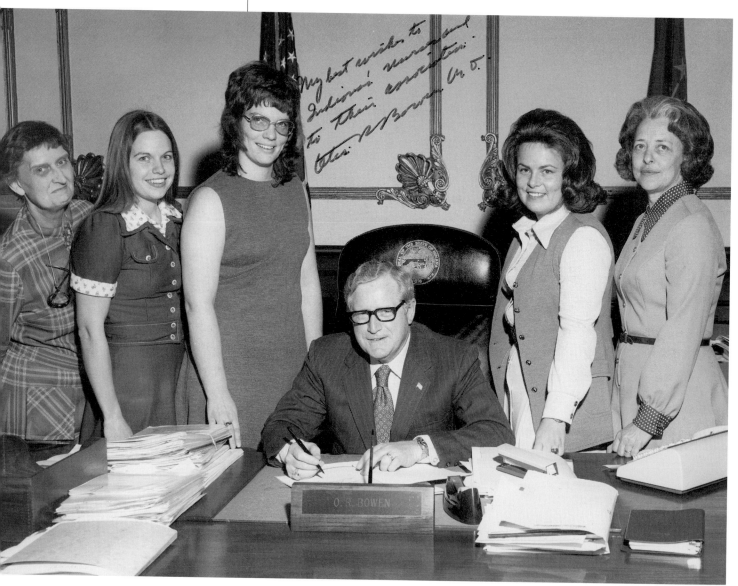

on in terms of what nursing's social mandate was. But at the same time, it meant that nurses would be and should be held accountable for doing these things."[54] The legislature passed the proposed definition in 1974, making Indiana the third state to pass such an act.

To implement the independent functions of nursing as defined by the new Nurse Practice Act, the ISNA Council on Practice developed Standards of Nursing Practice.[55] Although the standards were never put into the State Board of Nursing rules, their major importance lay in the fact that they could be used in a court of law as acceptable practice, for which the nurse would be held accountable. The ISNA was ahead of the ANA in developing standards of practice.[56] Consequently, when the ANA adopted its own standards at a later date, the national association used some of the ISNA language.

Indiana State Nurses Association staff in 1977 (ISNA Collection M0380, Indiana Historical Society)

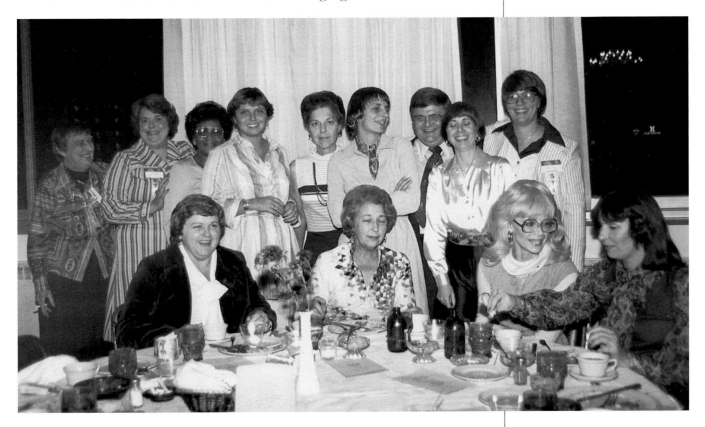

Endnotes

[1] Philip Kalisch and Beatrice Kalisch, *The Advance of American Nursing*, 3rd ed. (Philadelphia: J. B. Lippincott Company, 1995), 445.

[2] "Mr. C. D. Is Pleased to Announce," *The Indiana Nurse* 24, no. 2 (1960): 18.

[3] "ISNA Committee Reports, Civil Defense Information Committee," *The Indiana Nurse* 26, no. 3 (1962): 21.

[4]Dorothy F. McFarland, "District 12," *The Indiana Nurse* 29, no. 3 (1965): 36.

[5]"Military News," *The Indiana Nurse* 29, no. 4 (1965): 21.

[6]"Military News," *The Indiana Nurse* 31, no. 1 (1967): 20–21.

[7]1967 "Military News," 21.

[8]Merrill S. Harrison, "Nurses at Pleiku," *The Indiana Nurse* 31, no. 1 (1967): 21.

[9]Karren E. Mundell Transcripts, 1966, M700, Box 1, folder 10 (June 24, 1966), IHS; and Eric Mundell, "Karren E. Mundell Vietnam Correspondence, 1966–1967 Biographical Sketch,"http://www.indianahistory.org/library/manuscripts/collection_guides/m0700.html (18 January 2003).

[10]Karren E. Mundell Transcripts, 19 February and 13 May 1967, M700, Box 1, folder 11, IHS.

[11]Kalisch and Kalisch, 405.

[12]"Professional Nursing," *The Indiana Nurse* 28, no. 1 (1964): 17–18.

[13]"ISNA Sixty-Second Annual Meeting," *The Indiana Nurse* 30, no. 3 (1966): 3.

[14]Marilyn J. Bourgeois, "An Approach to Maternity Nursing for Men," *The Indiana Nurse* 34, no. 4 (1970): 16.

[15]Ibid., 17.

[16]"Committee on Professional Nursing Practice," *The Indiana Nurse* 26, no. 3 (1962): 21.

[17]"Closed Chest Cardiac Resuscitation…Professional and Legal Implications for Nurses," *AJN* 62 (May 1962): 95.

[18]Lucille Wall, "Legal Aspects of Closed Chest Cardiac Resuscitation," *The Indiana Nurse* 29, no. 4 (1965): 26.

[19]Ibid., 26.

[20]Ibid., 27.

[21]"Joint Committee Reports, Indiana Hospital Association," *The Indiana Nurse* 29, no. 3 (1965): 24–25.

[22]"Joint Committee Reports, Indiana State Medical Association," *The Indiana Nurse* 29, no. 3 (1965): 25; and *The Indiana Nurse* 31, no. 3 (1967): 18.

[23]"Board Action," *The Indiana Nurse* 29, no. 1 (1965): 4.

[24]Kalisch and Kalisch, 465.

[25]"U.S. Surgeon General Endorses Nurses' Pay Drive," *The Indiana Nurse* 31, no. 1 (1967): 5.

[26]"AMA Supports Nursing Salary Raise," *The Indiana Nurse* 31, no.1 (1967): 6.

[27]Susan M. Reverby, *Ordered to Care: The Dilemma of American Nursing, 1850–1945* (New York and Cambridge: Cambridge University Press, 1987), 197–198.

[28]"Professional Organization vs. Unionism, ANA Statement," *The Indiana Nurse* 27, no. 1 (1963): 22–23.

[29]"The President's Message," *The Indiana Nurse* 31, no. 2 (1967): 4.

[30]"Economic and General Welfare Program, ISNA Moves Forward," *The Indiana Nurse* 31, no. 2 (1967): 6–7.

[31]"*AJN* Marks 60th Anniversary," *The Indiana Nurse* 25 (1961): 4.

[32]Roberta R. Spohn, "The Future of Education for Professional Practice," (New York: ANA, 1962), Box 27, folder 7, IHS.

[33]Kalisch and Kalisch, 420.

[34]"American Nurses' Association First Position Paper on Education for Nursing," *AJN* 65, no. 12 (1965): 107–108.

[35]Kalisch and Kalisch, 435.

[36]Lois C. Meier, ed., *A Study of Nursing Needs in Indiana 1973* (August 1973), Record in ISNA Headquarters, Indianapolis, IN: vii.

[37]Ibid., vii.

[38]Helen R. Johnson, "The History of Purdue University's Nursing Education Programs" (Ed.D. diss., Indiana University, 1975), 1–4.

[39]Kalisch and Kalisch, 445–452.

[40]Meier, viii.

[41]Ibid., 1–3.

[42]Ibid., 1–21.

[43]Johnson, 136.

[44]"Resolutions Adopted by 1979 ISNA House of Delegates," *ISNA Bulletin* 5, no. 6 (1979): 3.

[45]Juanita Laidig, Interview with Dr. Brenda Lyon, 27 May 2003.

[46]"Continuing Education, An Answer to the Education Gap," *The Indiana Nurse* 34, no. 1 (1970): 22.

[47]Juanita Laidig, Telephone Call to Belinda Puetz, 22 July 2003.

[48]"ISNA President Testifies," *ISNA Bulletin* 2, no. 4 (1976): 3.

[49]"Ad," *The Indiana Nurse* 25, no. 2, (March 1961): p. 1,515.

[50]"House of Delegates Report," *50th Convention of the ANA* (1976): 70; and "ISNA Biennial Convention Issue," *The Indiana Nurse* (1977).

[51]"President's Message," *The Indiana Nurse* 25, no. 6 (1961): 6.

[52]Brenda Lyon, *Nursing Practice: An Exemplification of the Statutory Definition* (Birmingham: Pathway Press, monograph 1983), 3.

[53]Lyon interview, 2003.

[54]Ibid.

[55]"Special Issue," *The Indiana Nurse 1973 ISNA Biennial Convention Issue*, ISNA Archives, Indianapolis, Indiana: 8–13.

[56]Lyon interview, 2003.

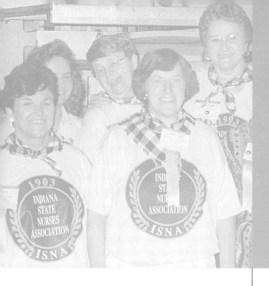

Chapter 6

"It's Time to Move On"
1980-2002

Marjorie Lentz Porter, Ed.D., R.N.

The September 1981 issue of the *Indiana Nurse* was titled "Moving on in the 80s." In her report to the membership, President Brenda Lyon issued the message, "It's time to move on!"[1] Dr. Lyon, who served as president of the ISNA from 1977 to 1981, no doubt was reflecting on the association's significant accomplishments during her tenure as president. At the same time, she was issuing a challenge to Indiana nurses that there was much more to achieve. Shortages of nurses, educational level for entry into practice, nursing's image, and low salaries were among the issues that continued to plague nursing during the 1980s.

"All the Buses Came"

Among the important accomplishments of the association during the 1980s was the Indiana General Assembly's passage of legislation for mandatory licensure for nurses in 1981. Until that time, the Nurse Practice Act provided title protection, which meant that only a licensed registered nurse could use that term or the designation of R.N. However, it did not prevent a person from performing the services delineated in the Nurse Practice Act as long as he or she did not represent himself or herself as a registered nurse. Mandatory licensure requires that only a registered nurse or licensed practical nurse may perform the duties and services defined in the respective nurse practice acts.

During the 1980 legislative session, the ISNA's leadership faced numerous obstacles in the process of passing this legislation. At that time, the president, executive director, and the chair of the Legislative Committee carried out the association's lobbying efforts. One obstacle arose when the chair of the committee hearing the bill asked for evidence of public support for mandatory licensure. President Brenda Lyon and Executive Director Linda J. Shinn appealed to the general public through television and radio appearances in support of the bill.[2] The community responded overwhelmingly, thereby convincing the Senate committee chair to hold a hearing. On the first hearing of the bill, hundreds of nurses arrived by bus from all over the state to demonstrate unity and support.

Two factors were particularly important in the passage of mandatory licensure legislation. First was the need to protect the public, and clearly this was foremost in the intent and the efforts of the ISNA. Secondly, the need to protect the public required a state agency responsible for the licensure of individuals and the regulation of educational standards. As a result of this legislation, the State Board of Nursing survived a process of sunset review that was occurring concurrently in the Indiana legislature.[3]

In 1980 the ISNA spearheaded the formation of the Consortium of Indiana Nursing Organizations (CINO). This was the first time that all known nursing organizations throughout the state came together as a collective body to address common concerns. In her opening remarks to the group, Dr. Lyon stated, "…We as leaders of a socially responsible profession must identify common and overlapping concerns for which we can unify and join forces while preserving the necessary uniqueness of each of our organizations and our right to disagree while respecting each other's positions."[4] The CINO was instrumental in the passage of the mandatory licensure bill, along with the informed nurses who came in buses and supported their profession and the ISNA. This collective of nursing organizations continues to be active in Indiana to the present day.

A New Home and New Leadership

In April 1980 the ISNA purchased the building at 2915 North High School Road, Indianapolis, for the location of its headquarters.[5] This move was significant because it gave the association a permanent home and visual identity. It also provided the opportunity to build equity and earn income from leased office space. The ISNA headquarters remains at this location today. Although the management of the property called for additional responsibility and work on the part of the staff, it proved to be financially beneficial to the association.[6] Between 1985 and 1987 a major renovation and redecoration occurred largely through the efforts of member Magdalene Fuller, and it improved the aesthetics of the environment and professionalized the workplace. Having a permanent home that was both physically appealing and financially viable was an important step for the association to fulfill its mission of serving its membership.

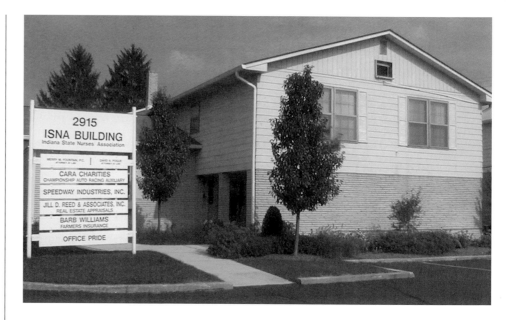

In 1980 the ISNA purchased the building at 2915 North High School Road, which has served as its permanent office and headquarters ever since. (ISNA Archives)

By mid-1984 staff leadership had changed completely. Linda J. Shinn, executive director, and Dr. Belinda Puetz, associate executive director, had both resigned to take new positions. The ISNA was without administrative staff for several months in 1983. According to then-President Dr. Sharon Isaac, she and Ernest Klein, Jr., who was serving as treasurer, kept the association going during those few months on "a wing and a prayer" until Naomi Patchin became executive director in September 1983.[7] In the spring of 1984 Ernest Klein, Jr.,0 was hired as associate executive director. In 1985 Barbara Carrico and Sara Denny became administrative assistants to provide essential support services for association programs. The association increased dues in 1983 and again in 1989.[8] It continued to grapple with issues of entry into practice, third-party reimbursement, and changes in the health care arena.

Strengthening Indiana Nursing

In the United States, health care costs continued to rise at an alarming rate, particularly in hospitals. Voluntary efforts toward cost-containment in the 1970s failed to control hospital costs, which comprised a major portion of total health care expenditures. In 1982 Congress passed the Tax Equity and Fiscal Responsibility Act, which altered the Medicare payment system from cost reimbursement of services to prospective price fixing using diagnostically related groups (DRGs) as categories for payment. As a result of DRGs, hospital admissions and lengths of stay decreased. This impacted negatively on nurse employment in hospitals. Emphasis shifted from in-patient hospitalized care to ambulatory care, primary care, and disease prevention. [9] In 1981 there were two health maintenance organizations (HMOs) and three free-standing ambulatory care facilities in Indiana. [10]

Acquired immunodeficiency syndrome (AIDS) was a new virus and little understood in 1980. The virus became a major health problem for the public, and infection control practices in health care institutions were radically altered as a result. An ISNA member served on an advisory committee for AIDS at the State Board of Health. In 1987 the ISNA addressed issues and questions regarding AIDS through guidelines for professional nursing care and safe working conditions. These guidelines protected patients and nurses by ensuring compassionate care, respect for confidentiality, and use of universal precautions. "How we provided for AIDS patients and protected ourselves in the process were two of the initial concerns," stated President Janet Blossom in 1985. [11] At the same time, the ANA identified AIDS as one of the ten issues of most concern to nurses. "AIDS is the most serious threat to the public health we have faced in a lifetime. We must do all we can to defeat AIDS on humanitarian grounds of decency and compassion..." stated Lucille Joel, president of the ANA, December 1988. [12]

Student enrollment in nursing education also decreased. The American Association of Colleges of Nursing reported a 34 percent decline in enrollment in Bachelor of Science in Nursing programs in the United States from 1983 to 1988. [13] The DePauw University School of Nursing closed in 1994 due to multiple factors, including decreased enrollment. [14] In 1995 there were eighteen baccalaureate, fourteen associate, and seven master's degree programs in Indiana accredited by the National League for Nursing. [15] The trend to close diploma programs continued with one remaining hospital-affiliated school in 2000.

In the midst of this period of change during the 1980s, the ISNA continued to advocate for nurses through constant monitoring of legislative action that could potentially impact the profession; collaboration with numerous health care organizations; provision and approval of continuing education; recruitment of new members; and improvement of the image of nurses and nursing in Indiana. In addition, the association continued to grapple with the issue of entry into practice. Since the first ANA position paper in 1965 that called for baccalaureate education as basic preparation for the professional nurse, this issue remained on nursing's professional agenda. An ISNA task force spent many hours developing a scope-of-practice statement delineating the technical nurse from the

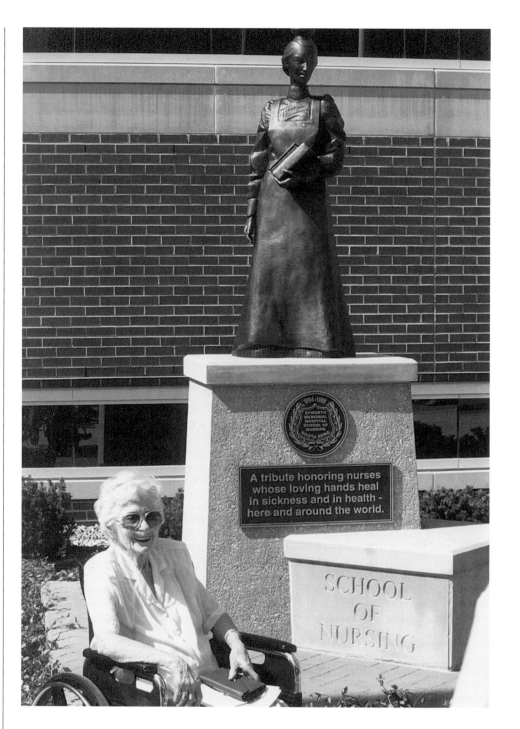

On June 16, 2001, Memorial Hospital (South Bend) dedicated a statue to honor its nursing school graduates. The facility, first known as Epworth Hospital, had a nursing school program from 1884 to 1998. Pauline Hammond, a graduate from the class of 1931, was present at the dedication ceremony. (Courtesy of Pat McQuade, Epworth Memorial Hospital School of Nursing, South Bend)

professional nurse. In September 1981 the task force published a comprehensive document titled *Future Educational Qualifications of Nurses*. A plan for legislative change was laid out; however, the division among nurses and lack of support from the health care industry worked against successful or meaningful change regarding this issue. Until recently (2003), North Dakota was the only state that required a baccalaureate degree for entry into professional nursing. According to Ernest Klein, Jr., executive director, the profession has been unable to come to a consensus on this issue and to articulate the differences in practice between levels of preparation. He stated, "Periodic shortages in nursing also contribute to reasons why we can't change the system."[16]

Another ISNA concern was third-party reimbursement for advanced practice nurses. Since the 1960s, the expansion of nursing roles occurred in response to the profession's increasing knowledge and skill base and rising health care costs. The roles of nurse practitioner, clinical specialist, nurse midwife, and nurse anesthetist were grouped together to form the category called advanced practice nurses (APNs). One of the barriers to the public's access to care was the lack of direct third-party reimbursement for the services of APNs. Thus, in 1985 the ISNA House of Delegates directed the Committee on Legislation to pursue the development and introduction of legislation for third-party reimbursement. As a result of the committee's work, it did not feel the need to mandate legislation but rather to work on "...strategies to facilitate the optimal use of existing mechanisms of reimbursement or to test the system prior to seeking legislative change."[17]

By 1989 federal regulations provided Medicare coverage for nurse practitioners in skilled nursing facilities, and by 1990 coverage included nurse practitioners and clinical nurse specialists in rural areas. A major victory for nurses and health care consumers occurred in 1998 when Medicare began to reimburse for services provided by nurse practitioners and clinical nurse specialists regardless of geographic area or practice setting. Many private insurance companies then followed suit. According to former President Dr. Ann Marriner-Tomey, the ISNA's legislative activities in the 1980s and 1990s were among the most important tasks the association undertook.[18]

To Organize or <u>NOT</u>

As noted in Chapter 5, Indiana nurses historically have never been heavily involved with collective bargaining. All of the states surrounding Indiana, however, have active collective bargaining units represented by their state associations, and some have been quite contentious.[19] The ISNA had one bargaining unit during this era in Marion, Indiana, at the Veterans Administration Medical Center. This unit was decertified in February 1986 when the employees voted to be represented by the American Federation of Government Employees of the AFL-CIO.[20] Later, the ISNA entered into an agreement with the Ohio Nurses Association to represent Indiana nurses.

A survey of nurses in 1984 indicated that there was support for collective bargaining, but the respondents did not want the ISNA to initiate organizing activity.[21] At the time of this writing, there are no active collective bargaining units of nurses represented by the ISNA in Indiana. According to Ernest Klein, Jr., who at that time was associate executive director, "One of the difficulties is that Indiana is an 'employ at will' state," which means that nurses (employees) can be hired and fired at the discretion of the employer without cause.[22] It also takes commitment and considerable amounts of time and energy to organize a unit. Indiana is a conservative state without a strong history of unions. The position of the association was and is to support and assist nurses who desire to organize.

"Thou Shalt Not Punish":
The Peer Review and Assistance Program for Registered Nurses

Guided by the leadership of Jane Meier, Denise Busch, and many others, the ISNA initiated the nationally recognized Peer Review and Assistance Program for Registered Nurses in May 1984 after two and a half years of planning by the Impaired Nurse Subcommittee of the Psychiatric/Mental Health Nursing Council and the Peer Assistance Program Implementation Committee. The underlying philosophical basis for this program was that nurses who were impaired by chemical dependency could be rehabilitated and should not be punished without being given a chance for recovery. Goals included: 1) to improve the level of nursing care to the public; 2) to educate nurses, managers, and the public about chemical dependency; and 3) to work with individuals who had direct or indirect involvement with chemically dependent nurses.

This was a tremendous undertaking given that volunteers composed of ISNA members provided it all. These volunteers spent many hours supporting and monitoring nurses who were involved in the program. In 1987 the Peer Review and Assistance Committee reported 100 referrals and 35 nurses in the program.[23] By 1991 the committee had received more than 275 referrals since inception, and it had monitored 60 to 65 active cases.[24] The Peer Review and Assistance Program continued until 1995 when the Indiana Board of Nursing took responsibility with a state-mandated program. For its duration, the program improved the quality of life for hundreds of nurses and ultimately improved the quality of nursing care of those whom their lives touched.

Continuing Education Continues

As discussed in Chapter 5, the association supported the notion of mandatory continuing education for relicensure, but its heart was not in it. The ISNA was not convinced that the provision of mandatory continuing education was related to improvements in care or practice, as studies had shown in the 1970s. By 1999 a Task Force on Continuing Education determined that "no evidence was present regarding the impact of continuing education on patient outcomes or maintenance of nurse competency."[25] That stance did not diminish the importance of lifelong learning for the ISNA or Indiana nurses. The ISNA Committee on Approval sanctions all state programs for nurses as providers whether they are individual or organizational. The ISNA continues to be accredited as an approver of continuing education in nursing by the American Nurses Credentialing Center.

Relationships with the ANA

In 1983 the ANA changed its organizational structure from an individual member organization to a federation of constituent state nurses associations. The purpose was to decentralize association activities and strengthen the state associations. Initially the change put a strain on the ISNA board and staff who assumed activities that the ANA previously performed. Other implications of this change were that states had more input into national issues of concern to nursing, and the ANA gave greater support at the state level.

In 2001 the American Nurses Association held its national convention in Indianapolis. Some of the delegates, members, and staff in attendance included: Front row (left to right): Ann Marriner-Tomey, ISNA past president; Nadine Coudret, ISNA past president; Joyce Darnell; and Janet Blossom, ISNA past president. Back row: Naomi Patchin, ISNA executive director; Lucy Tillett; C. Hazel Malone; A. Louise Hart, ISNA past president; and Barbara Baker.

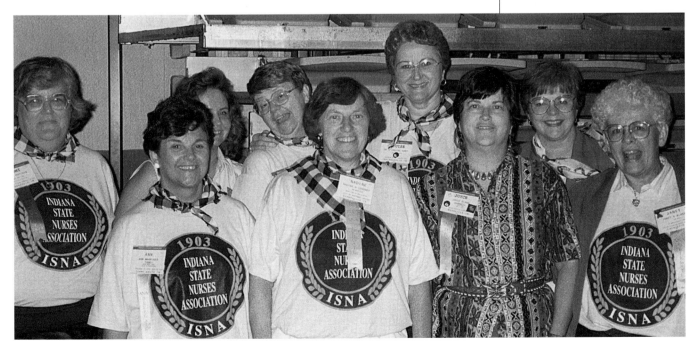

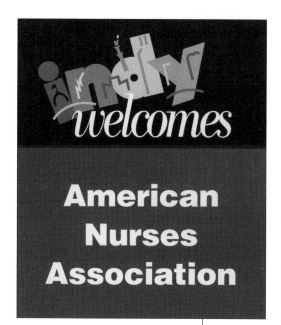

Indianapolis was the site of the 2000 ANA convention with ISNA as the host association. (ISNA Archives)

In 2000 Indianapolis was the site of the ANA National Convention. As host association, the ISNA was responsible for assisting in the implementation of this program for the large gathering of nurses from all over the United States. Dr. Charlotte Carlley was named coordinator, and with the help of numerous volunteers the 2000 ANA National Convention, "Keeping the Care in Health Care," went off without a hitch.

Computers Arrive! Technology Era Begins!

The impact of computer technology on the ISNA was significant in that it allowed for better, faster, and cheaper communication among members. In 1985 the association acquired its first computer, which linked the office with the ANA. The most frequently used computer activities at that time were word processing and internal office networking. By 2002 the ISNA had developed its own web site, www.indiananurses.org, hired Gary Abell as director of communications and marketing, and established electronic communication with all members who have e-mail.

The benefits of computer technology to the legislative agenda were numerous. The *Indiana Code*, which contains Indiana law, and previously was purchased in hardback form for thousands of dollars, became available online at no cost. The Indiana General Assembly can even be heard online while in session. Issues of the *Legislative Alert* are sent electronically, making them more frequent and accessible to members. The staff of the ISNA and the executive director monitor and communicate continuously to the membership any pending legislation concerning nurses' welfare and health issues. Since Alma Scott became the first executive secretary in 1924, the person in this position has looked for ways to communicate effectively with the membership. The association continues to explore ways to utilize computer technology for the advancement of its goals.

Coming of Age: Politics and Policy

Although legislative policy and action were primary activities of the association, the staff (director and associate director) and volunteers (president and chair of the Legislation Committee) performed most of that activity until the early 1990s. In 1993 the ISNA board established government relations—with an emphasis on health care reform—as a priority for 1994. The board also voted to employ year-round, part-time lobbying support.[26] The association hired SDS Group Ltd., a governmental affairs company, for a two-year term to represent the nurses before the Indiana General Assembly. Lobbyists Douglas Simmons, Glenna Shelby, and Ron Breymeier have continued working for the ISNA to the present day. This decision expanded lobbying efforts and liberated the staff and membership so they could focus on other aspects of the political process.

One of these aspects was the creation of the ISNA Political Action Committee, ISNA Nurse-PAC, in 1993. In concert with this decision, the Committee on Legislation supported the role of legislative district coordinator. These individuals were members around the state who had the ear of their respective state representatives or senators and could carry nursing's message to each and every legislator.[27] This network was developed through the exemplary leadership of Jodie Petrie, chair of the Legislative Committee. The ability to maintain these relationships continues to be a challenge due to the frequent change of elected officials.

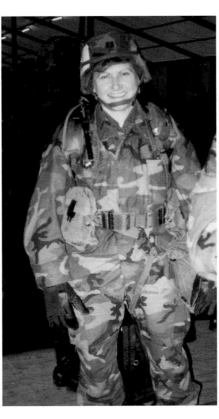

Anita Hupy Siccardi, ISNA member, served as a captain in the Army Nurse Corps in the Persian Gulf War from 1990 to 1991.

One of the functions of the ISNA-Nurse PAC was to endorse and support friendly-to-nursing candidates both publicly and monetarily in a nonpartisan fashion. Although Indiana nurses had a long history of legislative influence, they were new at financial backing and political endorsement of potential legislators. Fundraising, then, became a need, and the PAC directed its efforts toward ways to raise money for candidates. In 1996 it established a reverse check-off method of soliciting PAC contributions that would enable members to donate to the PAC along with their annual membership dues. In the first year of operation, the ISNA Nurse-PAC raised approximately $4,000 and developed an initial endorsement strategy for the 1994 election.[28] The strategy was to acknowledge, with endorsements and financial contributions, those incumbent state legislative candidates who had been important to the advancement of ISNA's legislative agenda. Of fourteen endorsements made, twelve candidates were reelected.[29]

By 1999 the ISNA Nurse-PAC continued to flex its political muscle. It made monetary endorsements to twenty-seven state legislators, all of whom were elected. For the first time, an ISNA member and practicing registered nurse, Representative Peggy Welch, D-Bloomington, was elected to the Indiana General Assembly. In 2000 the PAC endorsed twenty-nine candidates, all elected, with a total of $8,880 contributed to political campaigns.[30] One of the individuals most influential in the development of the ISNA Nurse-PAC was Jane Miller. In 1997 Executive Director Naomi Patchin stated, "Her selfless donation of time and effort has been invaluable in the growth of political activism within nursing in Indiana. The continuing growth of the PAC will be an ongoing tribute to her."[31]

Kaye Lani Rae Rafko, R.N., Miss America 1988, was made an honorary member of District 4 (in 1989) for her efforts to enhance and promote the image of professional nursing during her tenure as Miss America.

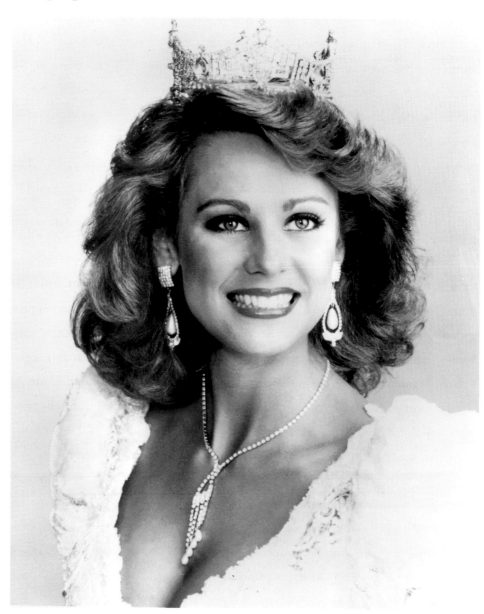

114

A Defining Moment: "The Nightingale Network"

In the 1990s the nursing profession moved aggressively into the primary-care arena where there was a void in care providers.[32] Studies emerged citing the competence of nurse practitioners and nurse midwives within their scope of practice as being equal to care provided by physicians. Around the country, nurses advocated for a loosening of restrictions on their practice, such as the need for physician supervision for diagnosing and prescribing, and the lack of third-party reimbursement. The AMA opposed such broadening of nurses' roles, contending that nurses wanted to practice medicine and not nursing. ANA President Virginia Trotter Betts challenged the AMA's assumption and argued that nurses were charting their own course. Maintaining that the bio-medical model was not the most useful way to provide health care, she explained that nursing would offer a new model, one that was more holistic in giving emphasis to wellness over acute, episodic care.[33] This controversy continued as legislators across the country began to revisit the role of nurses in the health care system.

In Indiana, however, a different picture was developing that was characterized by physician support. In 1993 the *Legislative Alert* proclaimed, "HB 1564 was approved by the Indiana Senate at 10:15 p.m. Thursday, April 8, 1993, by a vote of 49–0!"[34] This bill's passage was a significant moment for the association and the profession, occurring on the eve of the ISNA's ninetieth year, for it defined advanced practice nursing and granted such nurses prescriptive authority to prescribe legend drugs. Also included in HB 1564 were requirements for the Indiana State Board of Nursing to establish a program to monitor and support registered nurses and licensed practical nurses with chemical dependency. In reflecting back upon the passage of this legislation, Naomi Patchin, executive director at that time, gave much credit to the support of John (Chris) Bailey, M.D.[35] He served as state health commissioner and "provided eloquent support for nurses and the bill."[36] The efforts of many nurses were also instrumental in securing this legislation, and the term "Nightingale Network" was coined for their effort.[37] HB 1564 reflected a national trend that empowered nurses' roles in primary care and emphasized collaboration with physicians as opposed to supervision by them. One disappointment was that although the ISNA worked hard to help advanced practice nurses (APNs), the association's efforts did not bring more APNs into its membership.

Getting the Word Out

Publication of news, policy, and member activities has been a major activity of the association for many years. *The Indiana Nurse*, published biennially in conjunction with the state convention, serves as a kind of "report to the stockholders."[38] This document comprises the president's report; reports of councils; committees; task forces; summaries of the Board of Directors minutes; position statements; and public policy platforms. The *ISNA Bulletin* is a more frequent publication (four issues per year) that documents professional news of interest to members at the national and state levels, continuing education programs, offerings, articles, and advertisements.

In 2001 the Arthur L. Davis Publishing Agency contracted with the ISNA to publish the *ISNA Bulletin*, which is now distributed not only to members but also to all nurses in Indiana and to students enrolled in nursing education programs. The *Legislative Alert* is a subscription publication for members interested in or involved in the legislative agenda. It is a means of communicating the activities of the Legislative Committee and lobbying efforts to the interested parties. In 2003 the *Legislative Alert* became an online, members-only publication without charge and subsequently reached a larger audience. The online communication now includes requests for members to contact their representatives and senators on legislative issues pertinent to nursing. Members of the ISNA began to receive monthly issues of the *AJN* as a part of their membership package in 1996.

Advocacy: Surveillance and Support

One of the most important ways that the ISNA serves its membership and ultimately the public is through advocacy on issues that impact the nursing profession and subsequently the health of Indiana citizens. An example of its advocacy role was played out in 1989 when the AMA proposed a new category of bedside caregiver, the registered care technologist (RCT). The AMA offered this idea without input from the nursing profession as a solution to another nursing shortage. They stated that the RCT would be able to perform technical and bedside care activities under the direct supervision of physicians after completing a nine-month training program.

Professional nursing associations, including the ISNA, put up enormous opposition to the RCT proposal.[39] The association went on record with Resolution 1 to the 1989 House of Delegates to oppose the AMA initiative.

Fortunately, due to nurses' opposition and lack of public support, the entire RCT proposal was dropped and disappeared. As stated in the 1989 *Indiana Nurse*, Resolution 1 is an example of the type of advocacy stand that the ISNA typically took:

> ...WHEREAS, *Critically ill patients require more intensive and sophisticated care in a shorter period of time by caregivers who are more educated, not less; and*
>
> WHEREAS, *The introduction of registered care technologists would supplant nurses who are more educationally prepared than registered care technologists and who are already providing more comprehensive, direct nursing care at the bedside; and*
>
> WHEREAS, *The American Hospital Association has demonstrated that the registered nurse is the most versatile and cost-effective bedside care provider;*
>
> RESOLVED, *That the Indiana State Nurses Association work in partnership with consumers and consumer organizations to oppose the AMA initiative.*[40]

The State of the ISNA

By the mid-1980s there was growing concern about membership. Council and district reports in the *Indiana Nurse* throughout the decade are rife with the mention of the need for new members. In 1989 the membership was 2,256 out of 52,000 licensed nurses in Indiana, or only 4.3 percent. Annual dues rose from $185 to $205. There were twenty-one district associations covering the entire state. By 1995 total membership had dropped to 1,995. Numerous efforts were made to increase membership with no improvement. In 1997 the membership totaled 1,883. A Student Affiliate Membership project (SAM) began in 1997 and continues to be evaluated for its effectiveness in bringing in new members.

Partially in response to declining membership, the association studied its structure and that of other professional organizations who were experiencing similar problems and proposed a revised structure in 1999. The purpose was to streamline processes and maximize resources including the work of individuals. The primary changes were: 1) twenty-one district associations decreased to ten regions; 2) the size of the Board of Directors decreased and the officer position of second vice president was eliminated; 3) numerous committees were discontinued; 4) elected district delegates no longer voted; rather, each member would

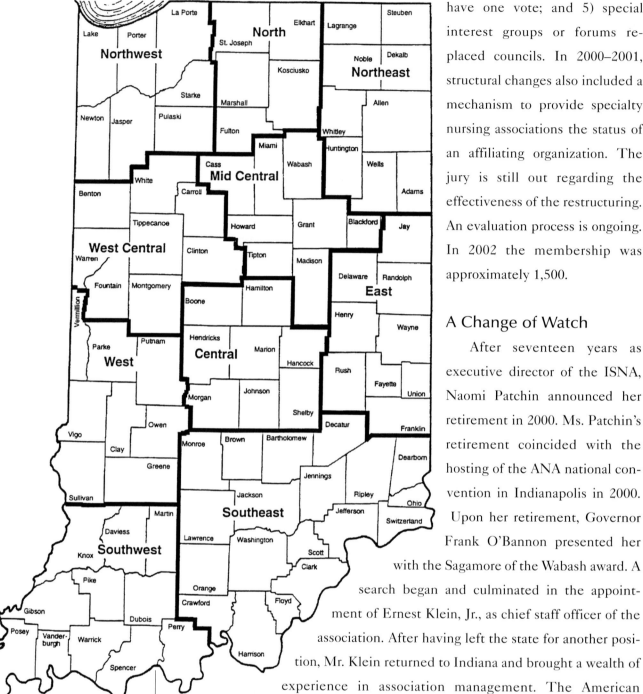

In 1999 ISNA reorganized from twenty-one districts to ten regions. (ISNA Archives)

have one vote; and 5) special interest groups or forums replaced councils. In 2000–2001, structural changes also included a mechanism to provide specialty nursing associations the status of an affiliating organization. The jury is still out regarding the effectiveness of the restructuring. An evaluation process is ongoing. In 2002 the membership was approximately 1,500.

A Change of Watch

After seventeen years as executive director of the ISNA, Naomi Patchin announced her retirement in 2000. Ms. Patchin's retirement coincided with the hosting of the ANA national convention in Indianapolis in 2000. Upon her retirement, Governor Frank O'Bannon presented her with the Sagamore of the Wabash award. A search began and culminated in the appointment of Ernest Klein, Jr., as chief staff officer of the association. After having left the state for another position, Mr. Klein returned to Indiana and brought a wealth of experience in association management. The American Society of Association Executives certified both Ms. Patchin and Mr. Klein as association executives.

Workplace Advocacy

With the appearance of AIDS, the constant shadow of health care redesign, and the nursing shortage, workplace advocacy became a major focus of the association's policy agenda from 1990 to the present. The 2001 state convention theme was "Workplace Effectiveness."[41] As nurses were being asked to do more with less, especially in hospitals, issues such as mandatory overtime, whistle-blower protection, unit reassignments, and sexual harassment were on the forefront. Workplace safety, not only in relation to AIDS but also with other infectious diseases such as hepatitis B, was evident in the 1990s both as a policy and as an advocacy issue. The association was united in its stand against smoking and alcohol and prohibited their use during convention sessions. After 11 September 2001, threats of bioterrorism affected health care providers,

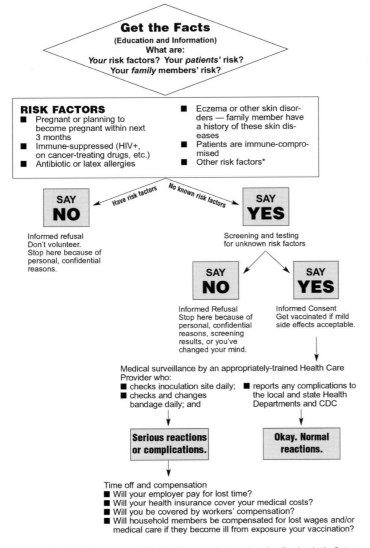

The American Nurses Association responded to the threat of bioterrorism in 2003 by offering nurses assistance in the form of a decision tree regarding smallpox vaccinations. (ISNA Archives)

including nurses, with concerns about anthrax, smallpox, and chemical agents. Advertisements in the *ISNA Bulletin* focused on factors nurses should consider before volunteering for risky procedures such as obtaining smallpox vaccinations. To many, the emphasis on workplace advocacy served as a substitute for unionization.

In summary, the ISNA's accomplishments for nurses and their patients in the last quarter of the twentieth century equaled in importance the achievements attained in the first three quarters combined. Among these were: 1) mandatory licensure, 2) a safer workplace, 3) help for the chemically-impaired nurse, 4) the election of legislators supportive to nursing, 5) support for continuing education, 6) third party reimbursement, and 7) prescriptive authority for APNs. All of these efforts have required much time, money and talent. While individual nurses in Indiana benefited by these accomplishments, it took the collective effort of the ISNA to make them possible.

———•———

Endnotes

[1] Linda Shinn, ed., "President's Report," *The Indiana Nurse* (1981): 14.
[2] Brenda Lyon, Interview by Juanita Laidig, 27 May 2003.
[3] Lyon, Interview.
[4] Brenda Lyon, "An Incredible Journey," *ISNA Bulletin* 28, no. 3 (2002), 9.
[5] Shinn, 16–17.
[6] Ernest Klein, Interview by Marjorie Porter, 23 April 2003.
[7] Sharon Isaac, Interview by Marjorie Porter, 10 April 2003.
[8] Ann Marriner-Tomey, Interview by Kathy Pickrell, 21 May 2003.
[9] Philip Kalisch and Beatrice Kalisch, *The Advance of American Nursing*, 3rd ed. (Philadelphia: J. B. Lippincott Company, 1995), 469–471.
[10] Shinn, 13.
[11] Janet S. Blossom, "Review of an Opportunity," *ISNA Bulletin* 29, no. 1, (2002): 14–15.
[12] Naomi Patchin, ed., "President's Report," *ISNA Bulletin* 15, no. 6 (1989): 1 and 4.
[13] B. D. Curry, "Societal and Marketing Influences upon Enrollment in Baccalaureate Nursing Programs" (Ph.D. diss., State University of New York at Buffalo, 1994).
[14] M. L. Porter, "A Case Study of the Organizational Lifecycle of the DePauw University School of Nursing, 1954–1994" (Ed.D. diss., Indiana University, 2001).
[15] *Nursing and Health Care* 16, nos. 2, 4, 5 (1995). Baccalaureate, associate, and master's degree programs in nursing accredited by the NLN 1994–95.
[16] Klein, Interview.
[17] Naomi Patchin, ed., "Committee on Legislation," *The Indiana Nurse* (1987): 24.
[18] Tomey, Interview.
[19] Karen J. Egenes and Wendy K. Burgess, *Faithfully Yours: A History of Nursing in Illinois* (Chicago: Illinois Nurses Association, 2001).
[20] Patchin, ed., "Staff Report," *The Indiana Nurse* (1987): 36.
[21] Naomi Patchin, ed., "Commission on Economic and General Welfare," *The Indiana Nurse* (1985): 13.

[22] Klein, Interview.

[23] Patchin, ed., "Peer Review and Assistance Committee," *The Indiana Nurse* (1987): 27.

[24] Naomi Patchin, ed., "Peer Review and Assistance Committee," *The Indiana Nurse* (1991): 37.

[25] Naomi Patchin, ed., "Task Force on Continuing Education," *The Indiana Nurse* (1999): 50.

[26] Naomi Patchin, ed., "Committee on Legislation," *The Indiana Nurse* (1995): 28.

[27] Ibid.

[28] Patchin, ed., "ISNA-Nurse PAC," *The Indiana Nurse* (1995): 54.

[29] Ibid.

[30] Ernest Klein, ed., "ISNA-Nurse PAC," *The Indiana Nurse* (2001): 43.

[31] Naomi Patchin, ed., "ISNA-Nurse PAC," *The Indiana Nurse* (1997): 37.

[32] Kalisch and Kalisch, 484.

[33] Kalisch and Kalisch, 485–486.

[34] Naomi Patchin, ed., "108th General Assembly, First General Session," *Legislative Alert* 13, no. 7 (1993): 1.

[35] Naomi Patchin, Interview by Marjorie Porter, 5 May 2003.

[36] Naomi Patchin, ed., "108th General Assembly, First General Session," *Legislative Alert* 13, no. 6 (1993): 1.

[37] Naomi Patchin, ed., "President's Report," *The Indiana Nurse* (1993): 14.

[38] Patchin, Interview.

[39] Kalisch and Kalisch, 477.

[40] Naomi Patchin, ed., "Committee on Resolutions," *The Indiana Nurse* (1989): 47.

[41] Klein, 2001.

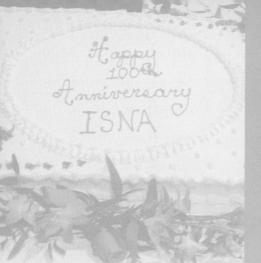

Afterword
2003-

In 1883, when Dr. E. F. Hodges concluded that nurses were due "respect and well-paid employment," he foretold of workplace advocacy issues the ISNA would address in the twenty-first century and likely beyond. At its 100th Anniversary State Convention, these topics remained at the forefront of the association's agenda. In the Plenary Session, Dr. Ada Sue Hinshaw, Dean and Professor at the University of Michigan School of Nursing, gave the opening address, "The Status of the Nursing Profession." Dr. Hinshaw was the first permanent Director of the National Institute of Nursing Research at the National Institutes of Health in Bethesda, Maryland. At the time of this publication, she served as Vice-Chair of the Institute of Medicine's Work Environment for Nurses and Patient Safety Committee. As a follow-up, she and a panel of representatives from the Indiana Nursing Workforce Development Group discussed the "State of the State – An Overview of Statewide Nursing Workforce Development." The following day at the Meeting of the Members, American Nurses Association President Barbara Blakeney also focused on workplace advocacy in her keynote address. As an expert in public health practice, policy, and leadership development, she was distinctly qualified to do so. Significantly, she discussed the current shortage of nurses and nursing faculty, and emphasized the important role of the professional association in lobbying for legislative action to meet this and other crises.

In addition to workplace advocacy, public health and education issues have continued to be a focus of the ISNA. At the centennial convention, members approved a resolution supporting public health nurses and their role in the public health arena. The ISNA resolved that it would advocate for: 1) competitive salaries for public health nurses, 2) investment in information systems technology, training, and public health nursing education to strengthen the public health infrastructure, 3) schools of nursing to include in their curriculum contemporary preparation for the professional public health nursing role, 4) an increase in the number of public health nurses serving in local health departments and other public health settings, and 5) certification of public health nurses.

A major concern for the ISNA continues to be its membership, which steadily declined since the 1980s. One of the contributing factors was the creation of specialty nursing organizations, which drew potential ISNA members into their ranks. These organizations were especially appealing because they were less expensive to join and they primarily focused on clinical issues of interest to nurses. Cultural shifts in the way people communicate and spend their leisure time also were important factors. At the centennial meeting, in response to a further decrease in membership following the 1999 restructuring, the ISNA members voted to appoint a task force to study issues regarding membership participation. The members also approved Bylaws amendments which will provide for expanded membership options.

In closing, Linda J. Shinn, president of the Indiana Nurses Foundation (INF), addressed convention attendees at the Foundation's breakfast. Titling her speech, "Unearth Your Brand," she emphasized that nurses identify their exceptional strengths and market themselves accordingly. She concluded:

> *All of us, each and every one of us, are perceived by others…for better or for worse. We are viewed each day as registered nurses, as specialists in our niches, education, practice, research, as ISNA and INF leaders, as colleagues, friends, spouses, significant others, parents, sons, daughters, citizens. And yet, many of us don't stop to think about how we come across or give conscious attention to the message we send…our brand, our identity, our trademark, our seal.*

> *Unearthing and managing our brand is not a selfish effort…it is an undertaking we should be engaged in for ourselves, our profession, and those we serve. It will make a difference not only in how we feel about ourselves but how we are perceived by our clients, and, perhaps most importantly, the viability of our profession, how attractive we are to the women and men we want to take our places.*

Linda J. Shinn, CAE

18 October 2003

As "inheritors of a great tradition," it seems fitting to conclude this centennial history with her challenge. Humility has its place in human affairs, but too often it is equated with passivity and weakness. If nursing and nurses are to be heard, we cannot afford to be timid. As the people in the ISNA's history have shown, advocacy is not for the faint of heart, but for the bold.

The 2003 convention had a record number of sponsors, exhibitors and advertisers. Their interest and strong support helped to make the 100th anniversary convention a great success.

Platinum Sponsor
Clarian Health Partners (clarian.org)

Gold Sponsors
Arthur L. Davis Publishing Agency (aldpub.org)
Indiana University School of Nursing (nursing.iupui.edu)
Indiana University School of Nursing Alumni Association (nursing.iupui.edu/alumni)

Abbott Laboratories (abbott.com)
ADVANCE Newsmagazines (advanceweb.com)
Association of Operating Room Nurses (aorn.org/chapters)
Community Health Network (ehealthindiana.com)
Ent & Imler CPA Group (eicpa.com)
GlaxoSmithKline (gsk.com)
Indiana Health Professions Bureau (in.gov/hpb)
Indiana League for Nursing (nln.org/stateleagues)
Indiana Nurses Foundation (indiananurses.org/about/foundation)
Indiana Organ Procurement Organization (iopo.org)
Indiana State Department of Health (state.in.us/isdh)
Indiana State Nurses Assistance Program (in.gov/hpb/boards/isbn/messages.html)
Indiana University - Purdue University Fort Wayne Department of Nursing (ipfw.edu/hsc_nur)
Indiana Wesleyan University (indwes.edu/academics/divisions/nursing)
Law Office of LaTonia Denise Wright, R.N. (nursing-jurisprudence.com)
Lutheran Health Network (lutheranhealthnetwork.com/)
Marian College (marian.edu/Departments_nursing.asp)
Marion General Hospital (mgh.net)
MARSH Affinity Group Services (seaburychicago.com)
MBNA America Bank (mbna.com)
Nursing 2000 and Nursing 2000 North Central (nursing2000inc.org)
Ortho-McNeil Women's Healthcare (orthoevra.com)
Parkview Health (parkview.com)
PEL/VIP (pulmonaryexchange.com)
Purdue University Calumet - School of Nursing (calumet.purdue.edu/nursing)
Roudebush VA Medical Center (appc1.va.gov/sta/guide/facility)
Select Specialty Hospital (selectmedicalcorp.com)
Sigma Theta Tau - Xi Nu At-Large Chapter (sf.edu/nursing/xinu.htm)
United States Army Healthcare (healthcare.goarmy.com)
United States Naval Reserve (navalreserve.com)
University of Indianapolis (nursing.uindy.edu)
University of Saint Francis (sf.edu/nursing)
University of Southern Indiana (health.usi.edu)
University of St. Francis (stfrancis.edu)

2003 ISNA State Convention Attendees

Esther Acree, Brazil
Dorene Albright, Griffith
Louise Anderson, Terre Haute
Donald Andrews
Kathryn Arnold, Carmel
Karla Backer, Indianapolis
Judy Barbeau, Hanover
Gloria Barger, Indianapolis
Peggy Barksdale, Indianapolis
Sarah Beckman, Monroeville
Carla Beres, South Bend
Doris Blaney, Hobart
Janet Blossom, Lafayette
Billie Bond, Greenwood
Jo Brooks, West Lafayette
Janie Canty-Mitchell, Indianapolis

Ellen Chesnut, Columbus
Kelly Christian, Cincinnati, Ohio
Elizabeth Ciyou-Allee, Indianapolis
Kathy Clark, Ossian
Nadine Coudret, Evansville
Elaine Cowen, New Haven
Wilma Cox, Fort Wayne
Nancy Crigger, Lafayette
Bonnie Culver, New Castle
Joyce Darnell, Rushville
Teri Davis, Fort Wayne
Colleen DeTurk, West Lafayette
Catherine Duchovic, Fort Wayne
Marsha Dyer, Washington
Judith Eichanauer, Decatur
Viann Ellsworth, New Haven

Patricia Erdman, Columbia City
Sandra Fights, Lafayette
Michael Fights, Lafayette
Opal Freiburger, Ossian
Connie Freiburger-Ashton, Uniondale
Jane Fry, Rushville
Sue Gaebler, Indianapolis
Nancy Gemmer, Fort Wayne
Jane Gordon, Crown Point
Linda Graham, Fort Wayne
Veda Gregory, Terre Haute
Carol Greulich, Columbia City
Linda Harbour, Terre Haute
Sanna Harges, Fort Wayne
Ella Harmeyer, South Bend
Ann Helm, Convoy, Ohio
Mervin Helmuth, Goshen
Teresa Holland, Greenfield
Margaret Housley, West Lafayette
Paulette Humphries, Richmond
Joan Hunt, Plymouth
Sharon Isaac, Indianapolis
Elizabeth Jackson, Indianapolis
Pamella Jahnke, Indianapolis
Karen James, Goshen
Carol Sue Johnson, Fort Wayne
Susan Kaiser, Logansport
Joan Kern, Fort Wayne
Linda Kerr, Fort Wayne
Joyce Krothe, Bloomington
Juanita Laidig, Greenwood
Janice Lee, Jasper
Karen Lothamer, Fort Wayne
Brenda Lyon, Indianapolis
N. Jean Macdonald, Indianapolis
Jane Manning, Indianapolis
Valerie Markley, Bloomington
Ann Marriner-Tomey, Terre Haute
Cheryl Martin, Goshen
Dana Mason, West Lafayette
Paula McAfee, Indianapolis
Marcia McCormack, Fort Wayne
Deborah McKibben, Washington
Susan McRoberts, Beech Grove
Linda Meyer, Fort Wayne
Barbara Mitchell, Carmel
Anne Moon, Indianapolis
Cindi Moon, Indianapolis
Michelle Morgan, Cambridge City
Kathy Morrical, Logansport
Kelley Murphy, Indianapolis
Donna Myers, Bloomington
Leslie Oleck, Indianapolis
Roselle Partridge, Indianapolis
Naomi Patchin, Indianapolis
Marian Pettengill, Indianapolis
Veronica Philbin, Cicero
Kathleen Pickrell, Terre Haute
Sandra Piercy, Shelbyville
Gloria Plascak, Terre Haute
Marjorie Porter, Martinsville
Sherry Rankin, Centerville
Beverly Richards, Fishers
Mary Beth Riner, Indianapolis
Brenda Rocha, Chesterton

Sally Roush, Frankfort
Donna Russell-Brown, Crown Point
Peggy Ryan, Bloomington
Lucinda Scheib, Fort Wayne
Barbara Schulz, Marion
Lee Schwecke, Indianapolis
Lou Ellen Sears, Indianapolis
Ruth Shearer, South Bend
Linda J. Shinn, Indianapolis
Melissa Spanburg, Bloomington
Cheryl Speikes, Marion
Phyllis Stanford, Hammond
Ruth Stanley, Indianapolis
Carol Sternberger, Fort Wayne
Elizabeth Stockdell, Charlestown
Diana Sullivan, Greenwood
Cheryl Switzer, Middletown
Sue Symonds, Kokomo
Jennifer Szabo, Portage
Martha Thomas, Evansville
Roberta Tierney, Angola
Susan Tossey, Indianapolis
Carolyn Tungate, Danville
Susan Vander Baan, Whitensville,
    Massachusetts
Catherine Vanderpool, Greenfield
Patricia Vaughn, Fishers
Cheryl Vines-Crooks, Chicago, Illinois
Jane Walker, Schererville
Susan Walker, South Bend
Clarice Warrick, Richmond
Joan Weber, Fort Wayne
Ann White, Evansville
Stephanie Whittaker, Indianapolis
Betty B. Williams, Lawrence, Kansas
Sandra Wood, Indianapolis

Convention Guests

Donna Boland, Indianapolis
A. Louise Hart, Jackson, Missouri
Elizabeth Hart Helms, Winchester
Belinda E. Puetz, Pensacola, Florida
Gary P. Dillon, MD, Indiana State Senator,
    Columbia City
Glenna Shelby, Indianapolis
Ronald Downs, M.D., Elkhart, President-
    Indiana State Medical Association
Karen Nichols, Elkhart
Ronald Wuensch, Executive Director, Indiana
    Optometric Association
Jim Leich, President, Indiana Association of
    Homes and Services for the Aging
Mike Wolf, Indianapolis
Laurie Peters, President, Indiana State Board
    of Nursing
Alan Peters, Kokomo
Kristen Kelly, Board Director, Indiana State
    Board of Nursing
Frankie Whitesel, Markleville
Timothy Whitesel, Markleville
Debbie Fights, Lafayette
Jennie Fights, Lafayette
Virginia Cox
Paul Cox

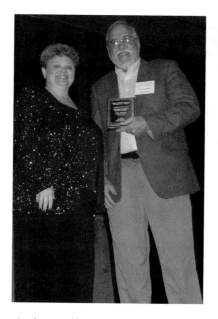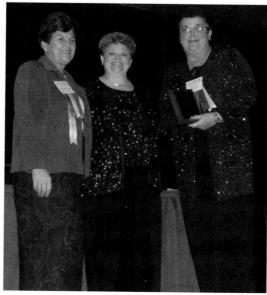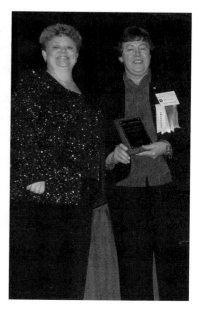

Goshen College, Indiana State University and the University of Indianapolis were the first recipients of the Nursing Education Program Recognition Award. This honor is bestowed upon the state's schools of nursing which advance the nursing profession by encouraging participation in professional organizations. At each of these schools the dean and at least 75 percent of the faculty are members of the ISNA.

Pictured in the three photos above with President Sandy Fights (left to right): Mervin Helmuth from Goshen College School of Nursing; Ann Marriner-Tomey and Esther Acree from Indiana State University School of Nursing; and Sharon Isaac, Dean, University of Indianapolis School of Nursing.

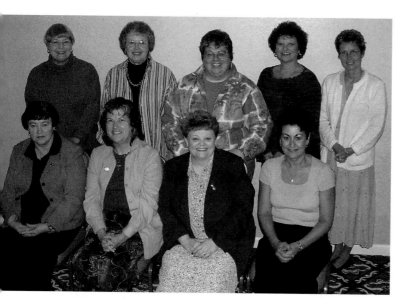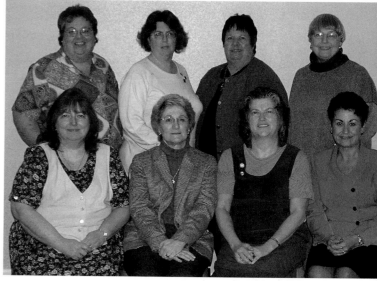

Presiding over the 100th anniversary convention were members of the 2001-2003 ISNA Board of Directors. Front row (left to right): Sharon Isaac, treasurer; Joyce Darnell, vice president; Sandy Fights, president; Dorene Albright, secretary. Back row: Directors Martha Thomas, Lou Ellen Sears, Ella Harmeyer, Veda Gregory, and Bonnie Culver.

The newly-elected ISNA Board of Directors held their first meeting on Saturday, October 18, at the conclusion of the convention. Front row (left to right): Terre Holland, director; Sue Gaebler, secretary; Joyce Darnell, president; Dorene Albright, vice president. Back row: Ella Harmeyer, director; Cindi Moon, treasurer; Judy Barbeau, director; and Martha Thomas, director. Not pictured: Barbara Kelly, director.

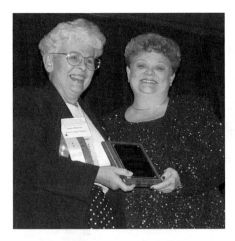 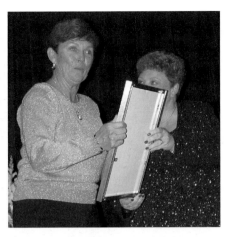 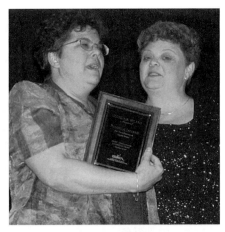

Janet Blossom received the President's Award from Sandy Fights. She was recognized for her contributions as a mentor and supporter of the association.

Beverly Richards received the Honorary Recognition Award.

Pam Jahnke was presented with the Georgia B. Nyland Award for her contributions to health policy.

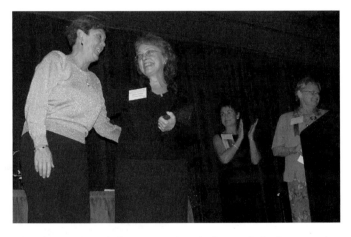 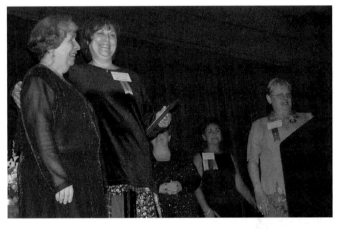

Beverly Richards (left) congratulated Ellen Eichel Chesnut who was the recipient of the Beverly Richards Psychiatric Clinical Nurse Specialist Award. The psychiatric/mental health special interest forum added Richards' name to the award to recognize her outstanding contributions to this specialty.

Frankie Lane Whitesel (second from left) received the Ruth Stanley Psychiatric Nurse Award for her work in this specialty area. Members of the psychiatric special interest forum renamed the award to honor Ruth Stanley (left) for her many years of service and contributions to the nursing profession. Also pictured are: Sandy Fights, Dorene Albright and Lee Schwecke.

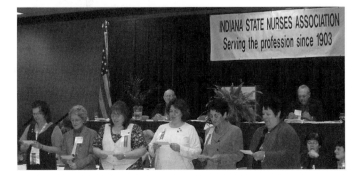 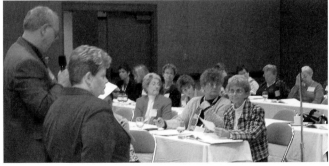

The 2003-05 Board of Directors took the oath of office during the Meeting of the Members.

Ernest Klein, Jr., ISNA Executive Director and President Sandy Fights reviewed many of the changes in the ISNA bylaws and other topics with members at the Issues Forum.

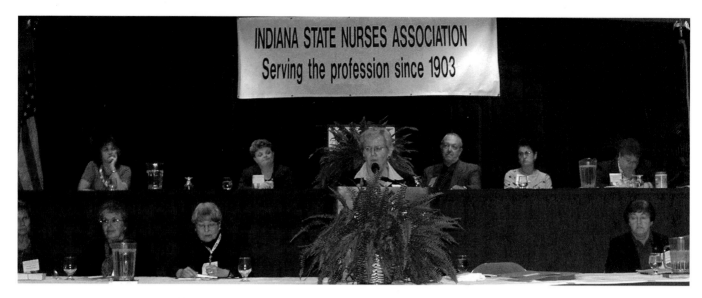

American Nurses Association President Barbara Blakeney delivered the keynote address during the opening session of the Meeting of the Members.

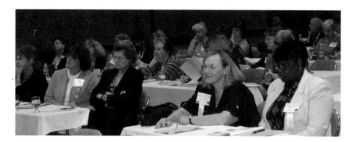

ISNA members filled the convention hall and listened intently to ANA President Barbara Blakeney's speech.

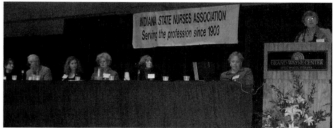

A panel presented information about the state of nursing in Indiana during the Plenary Session. Members of the panel included (left to right): Ada Sue Hinshaw, Bob Morr, Jr., Gwynn Perlich, Louise Neufelder, Jan Kirsch, Barbara Pantos, and Jan Bingle.

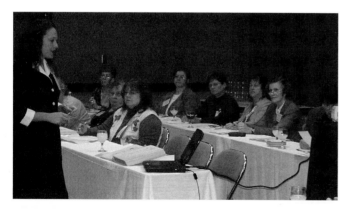

Erika LeBaron, M.S.N., C.N.S., R.N., presented a continuing education seminar on "Child & Adolescent Psychopharmacology Update." LeBaron specializes in child and adolescent psychiatry at the Midtown Community Mental Health Center in Indianapolis.

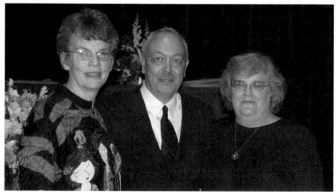

Former ISNA Executive Directors Linda J. Shinn (left) and Naomi Patchin (right) joined current Executive Director Ernest Klein, Jr., at the ISNA Awards Banquet.

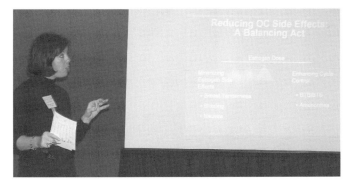

Julie Schnieders, M.S.N., R.N.C. and Nurse Practitioner, presented an "Update on Contraceptive Methods" during a continuing education session. Schnieders works with the Indianapolis Physicians for Women.

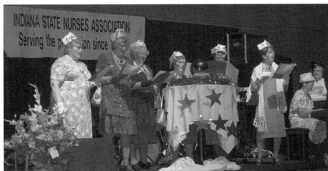

The Church Ladies, a comedy troupe from Fort Wayne, entertained the crowd during ISNA's Centennial Celebration. The ladies made "contact" with several famous nurses throughout history – including Florence Nightingale.

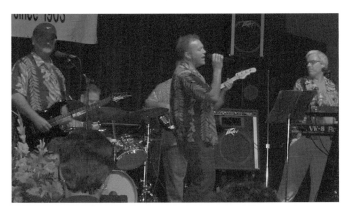

Frankie and the Bananas, a band composed of Fort Wayne-area healthcare professionals, entertained the hundreds who attended ISNA's Centennial Celebration.

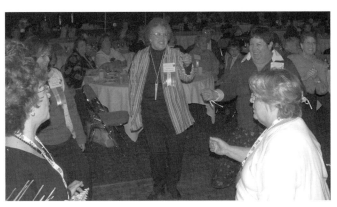

ISNA members danced to the beat of Frankie and the Bananas during the ISNA Centennial Celebration.

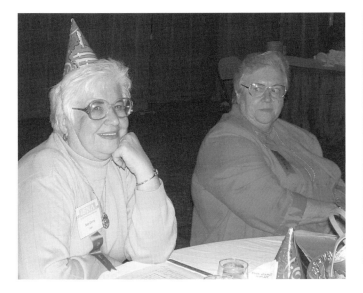

ISNA staff members Sara Denny (left) and Barb Carrico joined in the anniversary festivities.

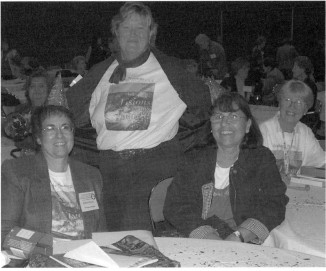

Left to right: Roberta Tierney, Sarah Beckman, Penny Leverman and Joan Kern enjoyed events at the Centennial Celebration.

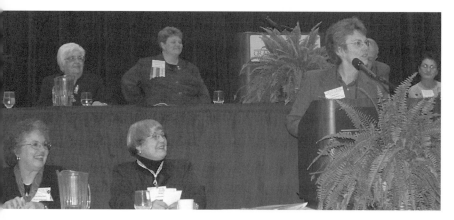

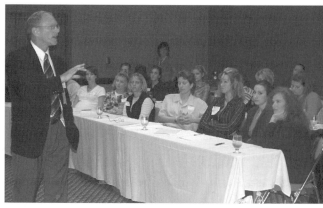

Linda J. Shinn, Indiana Nurses Foundation president, reported on the state of the foundation at the Meeting of the Members.

Scott Cleveland, from the Mental Health Association of Indiana, presented a popular continuing education seminar on the "Issues in Psychiatric/Mental Health Nursing Including Advanced Directives."

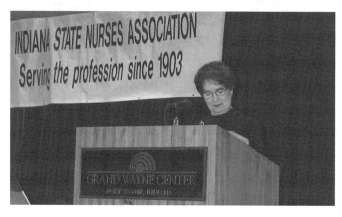

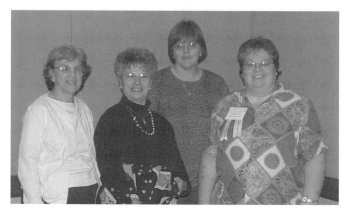

Ada Sue Hinshaw, dean and professor of the University of Michigan School of Nursing, presented details of research concerning the state of nursing in the United States at the Plenary Session on Thursday, October 16.

North Region members were contributing sponsors to this history book. Pictured here are some from the region who attended the Meeting of the Members. Left to right: Carla Beres, Ruth Shearer, Joan Hunt, and Ella Harmeyer. A complete list of North Region members is included in this chapter.

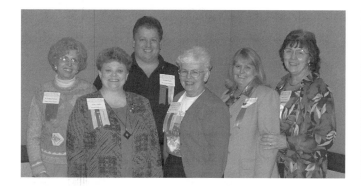

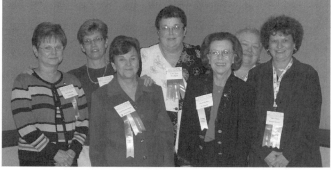

West Central Region members were contributing sponsors to this history book. Pictured here are some from the region who attended the Meeting of the Members. Left to right: Colleen DeTurk, Sandy Fights, Mike Fights, Janet Blossom, Dana Mason, and Peggy Housley. A complete list of West Central Region members is included in this chapter.

West Region members were contributing sponsors to this history book. Pictured here are some from the region who attended the Meeting of the Members. Left to right: Gloria Plascak, Kathy Pickrell, Ann Marriner-Tomey, Esther Acree, Linda Harbour, Louise Anderson, and Veda Gregory. A complete list of West Region members is included in this chapter.

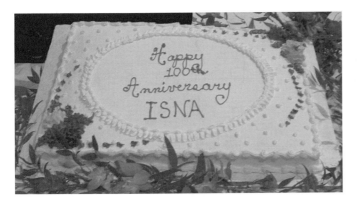

The special cake, marking ISNA's 100th anniversary, before members devoured it during the Centennial Celebration.

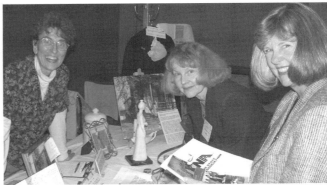

Pat McQuade, Margie Porter, and Jane Manning examined the many historical items that were on display at the Epworth Memorial Hospital School of Nursing Alumni Association's booth.

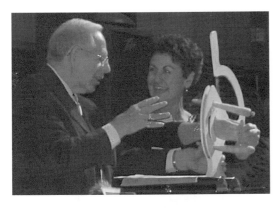

Magician Dick Stoner placed Dorene Albright's hand in a special cutting machine where he "guaranteed" she would not be injured. Stoner suggested she use her free hand to hold the one in the device just in case the trick didn't go as planned.

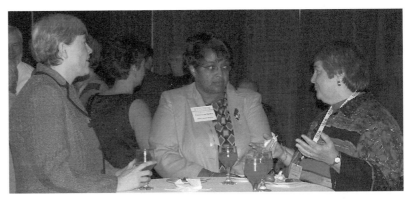

Left to right: Ann White, from the University of Southern Indiana, Cheryl Speikes, from Marion General Hospital, and Linda Graham, from IPFW, had a lively discussion during the President's Reception.

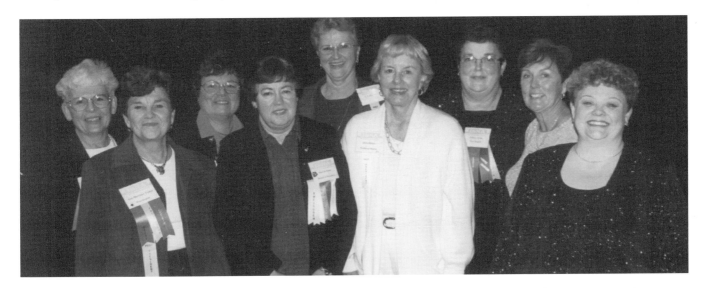

Several past ISNA presidents attended the Centennial Celebration. They include (left to right): Janet Blossom, Ann Marriner-Tomey, Brenda Lyon, Sharon Isaac, A. Louise Hart, Doris Blaney, Esther Acree, Beverly Richards, and Sandy Fights. Not pictured: Nadine Coudret.

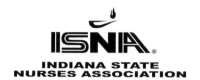

INDIANA STATE
NURSES ASSOCIATION

Presidents of the
Indiana State Nurses Association

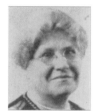

E. Gertrude Fournier*
Indianapolis
1904-1906

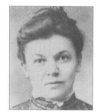

Edna Humphrey*
Crawfordsville
1906-1908

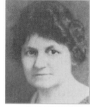

Mary B. Sollers*
Lafayette
1908-1910

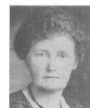

Maude W. McConnel*
Sullivan
1910-1912

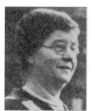

Anna Rein*
Springfield, IL
1912-1914

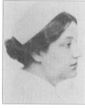

Ida J. McCaslin*
Lafayette
1914-1916

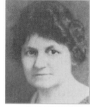

Edith G. Wills*
Vincennes
1916-1918

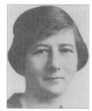

Anna Lauman Driver*
Fort Wayne*
1918-1919

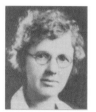

Mary A. Meyers*
Indianapolis
1919-1921

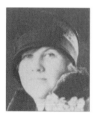

June Gray*
Indianapolis
1921-1922

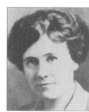

Ina Gaskill*
Indianapolis
1922-1924

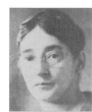

Lizzie Goeppinger*
Crawfordsville
1924-1926

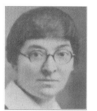

Anna M. Holtman*
Fort Wayne
1926-1928

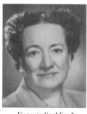

Eugenia Spalding*
Indianapolis
1928-1929

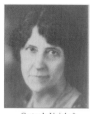

Gertrude Upjohn*
Indianapolis
1929-1931

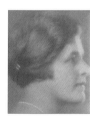

Lulu V. Cline*
South Bend
1931-1934

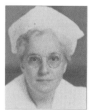

Nellie G. Brown*
Muncie
1934-1936

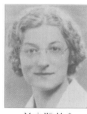

Marie Winkler*
Indianapolis
1936-1938

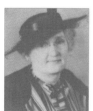

Edith Hunt Layer*
Terre Haute
1938-1940

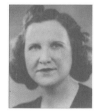

Anne Dugan*
Indianapolis
1940-1942

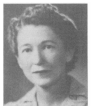

Mary York*
Bloomington
1942-1946

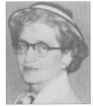

Nancy Scramlin*
Muncie
1946-1947 (resigned)

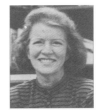

Leona Adams*
Indianapolis
1947-1950

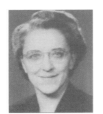

Helen R. Johnson*
Mooresville
1950-1952

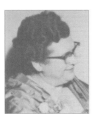

Helen Weber*
Bloomington
1952-1954

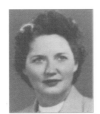

E. Lucille Wall*
Indianapolis
1954-1956

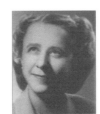

Genevieve Beghtel*
Indianapolis
1956-1958

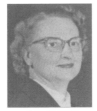

Florence G. Young*
South Bend
1958-1960

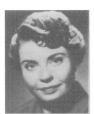

Dorothy Damewood*
Gary
1960-1962

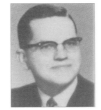

Marie D'Andrea Loftus*
Indianapolis
1962-1966

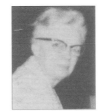

Richard O. Hakes
New Castle
1966-1969

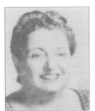

Emily Holmquist*
Port St. Lucie, FL
1969-1973

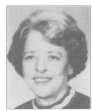

Jean Grimsley*
Madison
1973-1975

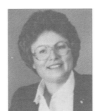

Kathryn (Lawson) George*
Indianapolis
1975-1977

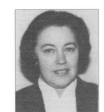

Brenda L. Lyon
Indianapolis
1977-1981

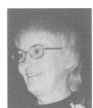

Sharon Isaac
Indianapolis
1981-1983

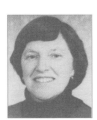

Nadine A. Coudret
Evansville
1983-1985

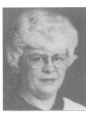

Janet S. Blossom
Lafayette
1985-1987

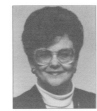

Doris R. Blaney
Hobart
1987-1989

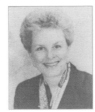

Ann Marriner-Tomey
Terre Haute
1989-1991

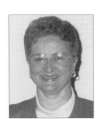

A. Louise Hart
Jackson, MO
1991-1994 (resigned July 1, 1994)

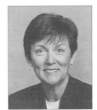

Esther Acree
Brazil
1994-1997

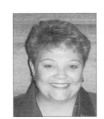

Beverly S. Richards
Fishers
1997-2001

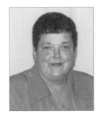

Sandra D. Fights
Lafayette
2001-2003

*Deceased

133

Thank you to the members of these ISNA Regions for their financial support of this publication.

North Region Members

Sue Anderson, Granger
Hisa Asaoka, Goshen
Joy Barnes, South Bend
Carla Beres, South Bend
Dawn Berger, Mishawaka
Edna Berkshire, Elkhart
Linda Bertsche, Goshen
Diane Biller, Osceola
Loreen Boggs, Fort Wayne
Nelda Bratcher, Goshen
Cynthia Brewer, South Bend
Linda Brock, Bremen
Fern Brunner, Goshen
Linda Chain, Plymouth
Ruth Davidhizar, Goshen
Carolyn Davis, Bristol
Carole Derucki, Niles, Michigan
Evelyn Driver, Goshen
Regina Drury, South Bend
Eileen Dvorak, South Bend
Diane Eldridge, Elkhart
Sally Erdel, Mishawaka
Loraine Fisher, Osceola
Ann Fitzgerald, Walkerton
Cynthia Fritz, South Bend
Patricia Gaither, Bristol
Rose Gesaman, North Webster
Deborah Gillum, Milford
Margaret Go, South Bend
Janet Goppert, New Paris
Peggy Grcich, South Bend
Tammy Greenwell, Mishawaka
Frances Grill, Elkhart
Elizabeth Gunden, Goshen
Ella Harmeyer, South Bend
April Hart, Goshen
Dawn Hatch, Elkhart
Mervin Helmuth, Goshen
Anne Hershberger, Goshen
Richard Hess, Middleburg
Kathleen Hoffer, South Bend
Wanda Hoffman, Goshen
Joan Hunt, Plymouth
Johnnie Jackson, Buchanan, Michigan
Karen James, Goshen
Rebecca Jellison, Elkhart
Diane Jones, Rochester
Douglas Jones, Niles, Michigan
Louise Jones, Elkhart
Catherine Junkans, South Bend

Joann Kaltenthaler, Kewanna
Dorotha Kauffmann, Goshen
Vicky Kirkton, Goshen
Toni Klatt-Ellis, Mishawaka
Sharon Klingerman, South Bend
Cathy Konecny, South Bend
Penny Krug, South Bend
Karen Kuklinski, Carmel
Beth Landis, Goshen
Judith Lee, South Bend
Arvilla Maier, Elkhart
Cheryl Martin, Goshen
Ulrike McConnell, Goshen
Betsy McCune, Syracuse
Tamara McNally, South Bend
Marian McQuade, South Bend
Patricia McQuade, South Bend
Lydia Meyers, Mishawaka
Amy Michels, Mishawaka
Barbara Miller, Syracuse
Denise Miller, South Bend
Elaine Miller, Goshen
Olive Grace Miller, Elkhart
Karen Mills, Rochester
Mashelle Monhaut, South Bend
Pamela Montgomery, Cassopolis, Michigan
MaryJo Morey, Granger
Debra Morin, Mishawaka
Kathleen O'Neill, South Bend
Judith Paton, Leesburg
Annette Peacock-Johnson, Granger
Katherine Penrose, Macy
Gretta Peterson, Elkhart
Margaret Pinter, South Bend
Beatrice Pyle, Elkhart
Phyllis Raber, South Bend
Beverly Rains, Espanola, Ontario, Canada
Janet Remington, Warsaw
Jacquline Richardson, Plymouth
Phoebe Ritter, Mishawaka
Kim Roberts, Granger
Colleen Rose, South Bend
Susan Rowley, Bristol
Kathleen Scarry, Benton Harbor, Michigan
Jayne Schellinger, Granger
Denise Scroggs, South Bend
Jane Seys, Logansport
Kathryn Shantz, Goshen
Laurie Shapiro, South Bend
Ruth Shearer, South Bend
Penny Shepard, South Bend

Barbara Shively, Etna Green
Cynthia Sofhauser, Granger
Barbara Springer, Goshen
Brenda Srof, Goshen
Helen Stackhouse, Warsaw
Stephanie Stanley, Elkhart
Susan Stelton, Niles, Michigan
Phyllis Syers, South Bend
Lisa Thompson, Elkhart
Dianne Tripodi, Plymouth
Laura Tucco, Chicago, Illinois
Crystal Underwood, Goshen
Debra Vance, Lakeville
Carol Vanwiele, South Bend
Christine Voorde, South Bend
Susan Walker, South Bend
Amy Wardlow, Elkhart
Mary Wcisel, Mishawaka
Joanne Weaver, South Bend
Mary Weber, Goshen
Norma Weldy, Goshen
Jeanne Wells, Greenville
Norma Wells, Rochester
Marcia Wenrick, Rochester
Cynthia Weyers, South Bend
Christine White, South Bend
Isabelle White, Rochester
Barbara Williams, Granger
Roxanne Wolfram, Granger
Beverly Wynn, Elkhart
Katherine Yutzy, Goshen
Linda Zoeller, Niles, Michigan

Southwest Region Members

Jill Alsman, Bruceville
Peggy Ball, Lincoln City
Jean Bandos, Columbus
Karen Bayles, Evansville
Virginia Begle, Ferdinand
Rita Behnke, Evansville
Ladonna Belangee, Mount Carmel, Illinois
JoAnn Belcher, Oaktown
Cathy Birchler, Elberfeld
Ruth Braselton, Owensville
Lois Brink, Princeton
Thelma Brittingham, Evansville
Deborah Brockman, Evansville
Rebecca Brunner, Mount Vernon
Norma Byrne, Princeton
Rose Carnes, Holland
Michelle Carson, Evansville
Jane Chappell, Jasper
Lillian Chappell, Evansville
Sheila Clark, Birdseye

Mary Anna Collins, Evansville
Nadine Coudret, Evansville
Cleo Cowan, Evansville
Kimberly Drennan, Fort Branch
Creole Dycus, Vincennes
Susan Dye, Evansville
Marsha Dyer, Plainville
Rebecca Elshoff, Evansville
Linda Evinger, Evansville
Rebecca Fehd, Evansville
Stephanie Fields, Newburgh
Vera Foley, Vincennes
Elisabeth Friedman, Terre Haute
Rita Friedmann, Vincennes
Pennae Fuchs, Evansville
Julia Georgesen, Evansville
Melissa Gilmore, Owensville
Margaret Graul, Henderson, Kentucky
Mary Haag, Loogootee
Shirley Haley, Haubstadt
Judith Halstead, Newburgh
Betty Harker, Tennyson
Deborah Harshman, Bloomfield
Sheila Hauck, Evansville
Wanda Hoehn, New Harmony
Peggy Hutchinson, Evansville
Patricia Jacobs, Bicknell
Leann Jochim, Dale
Karen Jones, Evansville
Lynn Jones, Newburgh
Lois Keerl, Evansville
Sue Keith, Evansville
Deborah Kinney, Evansville
Mary Kittinger, Evansville
Eleanor Lawyer, Washington
Roma Leach, Evansville
Janice Lee, Jasper
Robert LeVee, Mt. Vernon
Kathleen Lewis, Newburgh
Mary Lindeman, Huntingburg
Edna Lynch, Evansville
Pamela Majors, Evansville
Deborah Marshall, Boonville
Aleen Martin, Evansville
Cheryl McCarter, Vincennes
Judith McCutchan, Evansville
Deborah McKibben, Washington
Jennie McMahan, Vincennes
Vicki Meek, Odom
Judith Mefford, Evansville
Robert Mobley, Ft. Branch
Roseann Moody, Evansville
Judith Moore, Newburgh
Judith Morgan, Vincennes

Ann Motycka, Newburgh
Nicole Motz, Evansville
Barbara Neff, Washington
Charlotte Niksch, Evansville
Pamela Pepper, Newburgh
LaDonna Pfettscher, Evansville
Janet Plahn, Vincennes
Crystal Porter, Albion, Illinois
Angela Pruitt, Oolitic
Linda Pruitt, Newburgh
Joan Quante, Ferdinand
Robin Riley, Washington
Celia Rizen, Evansville
Susan Robinson, Newburgh
Marcheta Rodgers, Evansville
Mayola Rowser, Evansville
Jana Russell, Newburgh
Betty Ryan, Montgomery
Cynthia Schaefer, Evansville
Alice Schmidt, Richland
Dawn Schmitt, Owensville
Mary Schneider, Evansville
Maria Shirey, Evansville
Regina Sisk, Evansville
Dorothy Slaton, Evansville
Robin Smith, Newburgh
Julie St. Clair, Evansville
Gwendolyn Steyskal, Washington
Lynn Stiles, Evansville
Carolyn Stilwell, Evansville
Frances Stoll, Washington
Juanita Sullivan, Vincennes
Cheryl Thomas, Newburgh
Martha Thomas, Evansville
Mary Thyen, Jasper
Mary Toy, Newburgh
Linda Troutman, Montgomery
Karla Uhde, Evansville
Theresa Upton, Jasper
Beth Vincent, Evansville
Debbie Waters, Evansville
Elinor D. Weisman, Otwell
Julia Westmoland, Newburgh
Ann White, Evansville
Julie Whitsell, Evansville
Julia Wilder, Owensville
Betty Williams, Lawrence, Kansas
Katherine Yeager, Richland
Holly Yeatts, Newburgh
Marlene Yochum, Vincennes

West Central Region Members
Janet Ainsworth, West Lafayette
Alice Anderson, Dayton

Carol Baird, Ladoga
Kelly Basden, Lafayette
Marilyn Bell, Lafayette
C. Blanar, West Lafayette
Janet Blossom, Lafayette
Jo Brooks, West Lafayette
Margene Brown, West Lafayette
Trish Brown-Cordes, West Lafayette
Peggy Bryant, Chalmers
Chyi Chang, West Lafayette
Brenda Clayton, Garland
Suzan Cook, Lafayette
Cindy Cosgray, Idaville
Patricia Coyle-Rogers, West Lafayette
Theresa Coyner, Williamsport
Sara Craft, Cayuga
Nancy Crigger, Lafayette
Doris Crites, Otterbein
Marcia Daehler, West Lafayette
Colleen DeTurk, West Lafayette
Marsha Duda, Lafayette
Sharon Easterday, Lafayette
Ruth Ellison, West Lafayette
Michael Fights, Lafayette
Sandra Fights, Lafayette
LaNelle Geddes, Lafayette
Jeanette Goldsbrough, West Lafayette
Janet Hancock, Fowler
Terry Hancock, Fowler
Becky Hannowsky, Lafayette
Sylvia Hendershot, Templeton
Lela Hopson, Delphi
Margaret Housley, West Lafayette
Patsy Hoyer, West Lafayette
Vicky Hrdy, Lafayette
Gloria Huffman, Lafayette
Pamela Jeffries, New Ross
Judith Jezierski, West Lafayette
Debra Johnson, West Lafayette
Marla Kantz, Lafayette
Donna Kauffman, Buffalo
Jane Kinyon, West Lafayette
Stacie Klingler, Rensselaer
Sue Lazar, Zionsville
Jane Loeffler, Makowao, Hawaii
Judy Loudon, West Lafayette
Dana Mason, West Lafayette
Miriam Mathews, West Lafayette
Kim McDonald, Lafayette
Mary McHugh, Lafayette
Sally McIntire, Lafayette
Judith McIntosh, Mulberry
Tina McIntyre, Battle Ground
Susan McNett, West Lafayette

Jo Ellen Myers, Frankfort
Sharon Need, Frankfort
Kathy Nichols, West Lafayette
Julie Novak, Lafayette
Barbara Polstra, Lafayette
Sharon Posey, West Lafayette
Helen Pruitt, Lafayette
Gwyneth Pyle, Fowler
Anita Reed, Remington
Janet Rinehart, Hudson, Illinois
Patrick Robinson, Chicago, Illinois
Kathleen Schafer, Brookston
Pauline Schiavone, Oxford
Donna Schmeiser, West Lafayette
Genoia Segal, Lafayette
Linda Simunek, West Lafayette
Dianna Sneathen, Lafayette
Barbara Strasburger, Lafayette
Dianne Tao, Lafayette
Bonnie Trombello, Lafayette
Nadine Tucker, Lafayette
Deborah Villars, Frankfort
Emily Vonderheide, Lafayette
Jacqueline Walcott-McQuigg,
    West Lafayette
Candice Walker, Lafayette
Barbra Wall, Lafayette
Ann Webb, Delphi
Kay Webster, Lafayette
Debra Weirick, Flora
Kathy Whitaker, Lafayette
Sharon Wilkerson, West Lafayette
Ruth Wukasch, West Lafayette
Karen Yehle, West Lafayette
Anne Zahnke, West Lafayette
Mary Zink, West Lafayette

West Region Members

Esther Acree, Brazil
Meredith Addison, Hillsdale
Catherine Adler, Terre Haute
Louise Anderson, Terre Haute
Minnie Anderson, Indianapolis
Gloria Artigue, Terre Haute
Deborah Barnhart, Terre Haute
Renee Bauer, Terre Haute
Mary Bennett, Paris, Illinois
Diane Bingham, Terre Haute
Charlotte Black, Terre Haute
Jennifer Blank, Terre Haute
Dorothy Catlin, Terre Haute
Linda Drummy, Terre Haute
Leota Ehm, Terre Haute
Suzy Fletcher, Terre Haute

Paula Frank, Terre Haute
Connie Girten, Farmersburg
Veda Gregory, Terre Haute
Nancy Haggerty, Brazil
Linda Harbour, Terre Haute
Melody Hardway, Martinsville, Illinois
Tena Hedges, West Terre Haute
Ann Hendrich, Greencastle
Kathi Hill, Universal City, Texas
Maria Hockersmith, Terre Haute
M. Jan Keffer, Terre Haute
Jane Keyes, Terre Haute
Carolyn LaMar, Terre Haute
Debra Lambert, Terre Haute
Dawn Lee, Brazil
Linda Lewis, Terre Haute
Glenda Lopez, Waterloo, Ontario, Canada
Kimberly Mansfield, Terre Haute
Ann Marriner-Tomey, Terre Haute
Nancy McKee, Terre Haute
Helen Miller, Bloomington
Marcia Miller, Poland
Karla Monroe, Sullivan
Margaret Morgan, Cory
Whitney Morrill, Greencastle
Terra Mounce, Brazil
Dianne Nelson, Charleston, Illinois
Rebecca Norris, Carlisle
Dale O'Neal, Terre Haute
Rita Paitson, Terre Haute
Lisa Palazzolo, Rockville
Kathleen Pickrell, Terre Haute
Gloria Plascak, Terre Haute
Leah Ramer, Terre Haute
Sonja Rebeck, Terre Haute
Wendy Rowe-Perez, Terre Haute
Marilyn Sample, Terre Haute
Bonnie Saucier, Terre Haute
Susan Sharp, Marshall, Illinois
Norma Shaw, Terre Haute
Theresa Simon, Terre Haute
Lynette Smith, Clinton
Joni Steele, Brazil
Connie Steigmeyer, Terre Haute
Denise Stepro, Terre Haute
Sandra Thompson, Terre Haute
Donna Trimm, Terre Haute
Mary Von Leer, Terre Haute
Laury Wallace, Greencastle
Louwanna Wallace, Dana
Loretta Lucille White, Quincy
Susan Willock, Terre Haute
Connie Wycoff, Terre Haute

Chapter Contributors

Chapter 1

Kathleen Pickrell, M.S.N., R.N.
Associate Professor
Indiana State University School of Nursing
Terre Haute, Indiana

Karla Backer, Ph.D., R.N.
Associate Professor
BSN Program Director
University of Indianapolis
School of Nursing
Indianapolis, Indiana

Chapter 2

Barbra Mann Wall, Ph.D., R.N.
Assistant Professor
Purdue University School of Nursing
West Lafayette, Indiana

Chapter 3

Jane Manning, M.S.N., R.N.
Nursing Retention Coordinator for Methodist Hospital
Clarian Health Partners
Indianapolis, Indiana

Chapter 4

Diane Gorgal Eaton, M.S.N., R.N.
Nurse Entrepreneur
Fishers, Indiana

Chapter 5

Linda S. Rodebaugh, Ed.D., R.N.
Associate Professor
University of Indianapolis
School of Nursing
Indianapolis, Indiana

Chapter 6

Marjorie Lentz Porter, Ed.D., R.N.
Associate Professor
University of Indianapolis
School of Nursing
Indianapolis, Indiana

Indiana Historical Society (IHS)

Indiana State Nurses Association, 1887–1979, M380

Advisory Committee on Nursing to Letitia Carter, Director, Women's Work, ERA. Box 10, folder 13.
Advisory Council Minutes. Box 7, folder 3.
Annual Meetings of the Indiana State Nurses Association. Box 2, folders 1–13 (1903–1927); Box 3, folders 1–12 (1928–1933); Box 4, folders 1–12 (1934–1939); Box 5, folders 1–12 (1940-1947); Box 6, folders 1–13 (1948–1952); Box 7, folders 1–10 (1953-1956); Box 8, folders 1–12 (1957–1961).
Annual Meetings: State Office. Box 9, folders 1–11 (1919–1973).
"Articles of Incorporation." Box 10, folder 10.
"A Union in Indiana, Nurses Affiliated with the A.F. of L. Still Speak of Their 'Practice.'" 1910. Box 11, folder 10.
Brown, Sarah. "Report of the Chairman of the Legislative Committee." April 1905. Box 12, folder 9.
Cline, L. V. "The Present Problems and Needs of Indiana." October 1933. Box 3, folder 12. Code of Ethics. Box 20, folder 9.
Cox, Lizzie M. "Inspector's Report of Hospital Training Schools." 12 September 1908. Box 12, folder 9.
Dock, Lavinia to Miss Currie. 13 June 1910. Box 11, folder 10.
Foley, Matthew O. to June Gray. 6 May 1924. Box 11, folder 1.
"For Registration of Nurses." Box 12, folder 9.
Fournier, E. Gertrude. "How We Laid the Foundation of Our State Nurses Society in Indiana," written for the Twenty-Third Annual Convention of the ISNA. Box 12, folder 9.
"Indiana Nurses Will Demand Registration." 22 February 1904. Box 12, folder 9.
History of the ISNA. Box 12, folder 9.
Huesmann, L. C. to Ina M. Gaskill. 4 December 1922. Box 11, folder 1.
Johnson, Elizabeth. Memo Book. 1937. Box 12, folder 10.
McConnell, Maude W. Typed copy of Report. Box 12, folder 9.
McConnell, Maude W. to Miss June Gray, 20 April (no year). Box 12, folder 9.
Minutes of Graduate Nurse Association. Box 1, folder 1.
Nursing Councils for War Services—Correspondence and Papers. 1941–1945. Box 25, folder 9.
"Officers Elected by Nurses' Association." n.d. Box 2, folder 1.
Program, *Twenty-Fifth Annual Meeting, Indiana State Nurses Association.* 21–22 October 1927. Box 12, folder 10.
"Report of Chairman of Committee on Distribution of Nursing Service and Registries." 15 October 1933. Box 3, folder 12.
"Report of the Indiana State Board of Examination and Registration of Nurses." Box 5, folder 12; and Box 26, folder 2.
"Salient Facts for Ready Reference." Box 26, folder 2.
Schmoe, Delta. Document from the Nursing Service Bureau. 15 April 1935. Box 11, folder 1.
Scott, Alma H. "Indiana State Nurses Association." 1925, Box 12, folder 9; and 1926, Box 12, folder 10.
Spohn, Roberta R. "The Future of Education for Professional Practice." New York: ANA, 1962. Box 27, folder 7.
Teal, Helen to Miss Smith. 6 December 1933. Box 10, folder 13.
Teal, Helen. "What Was Accomplished in Public Health by CWA Nurses in Indiana." 1934.
Teal, Helen. "Final Report of CWA Nurses in Public Health." 1934. Box 10, folder 13.
"Trained Nurse Bill Has Narrow Escape." Box 12, folder 9.
Tudor, Nora. "Minutes of the 27th National Biennial Nursing Convention." Box 12, folder 10.
"Woman Wants Male Board." Box 12, folder 9.

Other Archival Sources:

Annual Report: Flower Mission Training School for Nurses, January 1890. Indianapolis: Reprint Marion County General Hospital, 1961.
Cecelia, Mother Mary. Diary, 15 May 1861. Archives of the Sisters of Providence of Saint-Mary-of-the-Woods, Indiana.
Hannaman, William. *Indiana Sanitary Commission: Final Report of Officers, 1866.* 18 August 1866. Indiana State Archives.

Meier, Lois C., ed. *A Study of Nursing Needs in Indiana 1973.* August 1973. Record in ISNA Headquarters, Indianapolis, Indiana.

Mundell, Karren E. Transcripts, 1966–1967. M700, Box 1, folders 10–11, Indiana Historical Society.

"Official Actions of the Catholic Hospital Association with Reference to Nursing Education." Archives of the Catholic Health Association, St. Louis, Missouri.

One Hundred Years Young—Anniversary Book 1878–1978 (Fort Wayne, Indiana: Parkview Hospital, 1978), Allen County Historical Society, Fort Wayne, Indiana.

"Special Issue." *The Indiana Nurse 1973 ISNA Biennial Convention Issue*, ISNA Headquarters, Indianapolis, Indiana: 8–13.

Newspapers:

Indianapolis Daily Journal.

E. F. Hodges's Letter to the Editor, *Indianapolis Journal*, Box 12, folder 9.

Theses and Dissertations:

Curry, B. D. "Societal and Marketing Influences upon Enrollment in Baccalaureate Nursing Programs." Ph.D. diss., State University of New York at Buffalo, 1994.

Johnson, Helen R. "History of Purdue University's Nursing Education Programs." Ed.D. diss., Indiana University, 1975.

Porter, Marjorie Lentz. "A Case Study of the Organizational Lifecycle of the DePauw University School of Nursing, 1954–1994. Ed.D. diss., Indiana University, 2001.

Schroder, Mary M. "History of the Indiana State Nurses' Association." M.A. thesis, University of Chicago. 1958.

Interviews:

Laidig, Juanita. Interview with Brenda Lyon. 27 May 2003.

Pickrell, Kathy. Interview with Ann Marriner-Tomey. 21 May 2003.

Porter, Marjorie. Interview with Ernest Klein. 23 April 2003.

Porter, Marjorie. Interview with Sharon Isaac. 10 April 2003.

Porter, Marjorie. Interview with Naomi Patchin. 5 May 2003.

Laidig, Juanita. Telephone call to Belinda Puetz. 22 July 2003.

Books:

Adams, George W. *Doctors in Blue: The Medical History of the Union Army in the Civil War.* Baton Rouge: Louisiana State University Press, 1952.

Allen, Dotaline. *History of Nursing in Indiana.* Indianapolis: Wolfe Publishing, 1950.

Barnhart, Deborah A., ed. *Caring for the Past and Future: An Historical Perspective.* Terre Haute: Indiana State University School of Nursing, 1988.

Barnhart, John D., and Dorothy L. Riker. *Indiana to 1816: The Colonial Period.* Indianapolis: Indiana Historical Bureau and Indiana Historical Society, 1971.

Blackwelder, Julia Kirk. *Now Hiring: The Feminization of Work in the United States, 1900–1995.* College Station: Texas A&M University Press, 1997.

Boyd, Louie Croft. *State Registration for Nurses.* Philadelphia: W. B. Saunders Company, 1915.

Egenes, Karen J., and Wendy K. Burgess. *Faithfully Yours: A History of Nursing in Illinois.* Chicago: Illinois Nurses' Association, 2001.

Eller, Betty Cotner, and Virginia Maier Cafouros, ed. *110th Anniversary of the Wishard Memorial Hospital School of Nursing.* Indianapolis: private printing by authors, 1993.

Esarey, Logan. *History of Indiana from its Exploration to 1922*, vol. 1. Dayton, Ohio: Historical Publishing Co., 1922.

Esarey, Logan. *History of Indiana.* New York: Harcourt, Brace, 1922.

Faragher, John Mack, et al. *Out of Many: A History of the American People, Combined Edition*, Brief 3rd ed. Upper Saddle River, New Jersey: Prentice Hall, 2001.

Hale, Hester Anne. *Caring for the Community: The History of Wishard Hospital*, Indianapolis: Wishard Memorial Foundation, 1999.

Hine, Darlene Clark. *Black Women in White: Racial Conflict and Cooperation in the Nursing Profession, 1890–1950.* Bloomington and Indianapolis: Indiana University Press, 1989.

Kalisch, Philip A., and Beatrice J. Kalisch. *The Advance of American Nursing.* Philadelphia: J. B. Lippincott Co., 1995.

Lewenson, Sandra Beth. *Taking Charge: Nursing, Suffrage, & Feminism in America, 1873–1920.* New York: NLN Press, 1996.

Logan, Sister Eugenia. *History of the Sisters of Providence of Saint-Mary-of-the-Woods*, vol. 2. Terre Haute, IN: Moore-Langen Printing Co., 1978.

Lyon, Brenda. *Nursing Practice: An Exemplification of the Statutory Definition*. Birmingham: Pathway Press, monograph 1983.

Madison, James H. *Indiana Through Tradition and Change: A History of the Hoosier State and Its People, 1920–1945*. Indianapolis: Indiana Historical Society, 1982.

Marriner-Tomey, Ann, ed. *Nursing in Indiana: 75 Years at the Heart of Health Care*. Indianapolis: Indiana University School of Nursing, 1989.

McPherson, James M. *Battle Cry of Freedom: The Civil War Era*. New York: Ballantine Books, 1988.

Melosh, Barbara. *"The Physician's Hand": Work Culture and Conflict in American Nursing*. Philadelphia: Temple University Press, 1982.

Moore, Frank. *Women of the War*. Hartford, CT: National Publishing Co., 1866.

Morrison, Olin D. *Indiana's Care of Her Soldiers in the Field, 1861–1865*. Bloomington: Indiana University, 1926.

Nutting, M. Adelaide. *Educational Status of Nursing, Bulletin #7*. Washington, DC: Government Printing Office, 1912.

Reverby, Susan M. *Ordered to Care—The Dilemma of American Nursing, 1850–1945*. Cambridge: Cambridge University Press, 1987.

Russo, Dorothy R. *One Hundred Years of Indiana Medicine, 1849–1949*. Indianapolis: Indiana State Medical Association, 1950.

Phillips, Clifton J. *Indiana in Transition: The Emergence of an Industrial Commonwealth, 1880–1920*. Indianapolis: Indiana Historical Bureau and Indiana Historical Society, 1968.

Stevens, Rosemary. *In Sickness and in Wealth: American Hospitals in the Twentieth Century*. Baltimore and London: Johns Hopkins University Press, 1989; repr. 1999.

Stewart, Isabel M., and Anne L. Austin. *A History of Nursing*. New York: G. P. Putnam's Sons, 1962.

Wishard, Elizabeth Moreland. *William Henry Wishard, A Doctor of the Old School*. Indianapolis: Hollenbeck Press, 1920. p. 278.

Articles:

"Ad." *The Indiana Nurse* 25, no. 2 (March 1961): p. 1,515.

Allen, Dotaline E. "History of Nursing in Indiana," in D. Russo, ed., *One Hundred Years of Indiana Medicine, 1849–1949*. Indianapolis: Indiana State Medical Association, 1950.

"*AJN* Marks 60th Anniversary." *The Indiana Nurse* 25 (1961): 4.

"AMA Supports Nursing Salary Raise." *The Indiana Nurse* 31, no.1 (1967): 6.

"A Membership Campaign." *AJN* 24, no. 13 (1924): 1,023–1,025.

"American Nurses' Association First Position Paper on Education for Nursing." *AJN* 65, no. 12 (1965): 107–108.

Ashendel, Anita. "'Women as Force' in Indiana History." In *The State of Indiana History, 2000*, edited by Robert M. Taylor. Indianapolis: Indiana Historical Society, 2001.

Blossom, Janet S. "Review of an Opportunity." *ISNA Bulletin* 29, no. 1 (2002): 14–15.

"Board Action." *The Indiana Nurse* 29, no. 1 (1965): 4.

Bourgeois, Marilyn J. "An Approach to Maternity Nursing for Men." *The Indiana Nurse* 34, no. 4 (1970): 16.

Christy, Teresa E. "Nurses in American History: The Fateful Decade, 1890–1900." *American Journal of Nursing* 75, No. 7 (1975): 1,163.

"Civilian Registered Nurses Needed in Viet Nam." *The Indiana Nurse* 30, no. 4 (1966): 9.

"Continuing Education, An Answer to the Education Gap." *The Indiana Nurse* 34, no. 1 (1970): 22.

"Coronary Care—Nurses Prepare." *The Indiana Nurse* 32, no. 4 (1968): 13–14.

Clarke, Ethel P. "Alma Ham Scott—Organizer." *AJN* 36, no. 2 (1936): 149–152.

"Closed Chest Cardiac Resuscitation…Professional and Legal Implications for Nurses." *AJN* 62 (May 1962): 95.

"Committee on Professional Nursing Practice." *The Indiana Nurse* 26, no. 3 (1962): 21.

"Decision Time in '79." *The Indiana Nurse 1979 ISNA Biennial Convention Issue* (1979): 1.

"Economic and General Welfare Program, ISNA Moves Forward." *The Indiana Nurse* 31, no. 2 (1967): 6–7.

"Editorials." *AJN* 24 (1924): 191.

"Grace Julian Clarke." In *The Social Register of Indiana*. Indianapolis: The Social Register of Indiana, 1912.

Harrison, Merrill S. "Nurses at Pleiku." *The Indiana Nurse* 31, no. 1 (1967): 21.

"House of Delegates Report." *50th Convention of the ANA* (1976): 70.

"Institute Considers Minority Problems." *The Indiana Nurse* (1957): 4–5.

"ISNA Biennial Convention Issue." *The Indiana Nurse* (1977).

"ISNA Committee Reports, Civil Defense Information Committee." *The Indiana Nurse* 26, no. 3 (1962): 21.

"ISNA President Testifies." *ISNA Bulletin* 2, no. 4 (1976): 3.

"ISNA Sixty-Second Annual Meeting." *The Indiana Nurse* 30, no. 3 (1966): 3.

"Joint Committee Reports, Indiana Hospital Association." *The Indiana Nurse* 29, no. 3 (1965): 24–25.

"Joint Committee Reports, Indiana State Medical Association." *The Indiana Nurse* 29, no. 3 (1965): 25.

"Joint Committee Reports, Indiana State Medical Association." *The Indiana Nurse* 31, no. 3 (1967): 18.

Klein, Ernest, ed. "ISNA-Nurse PAC." *The Indiana Nurse* (2001): 43.

Lyon, Brenda. "An Incredible Journey." *ISNA Bulletin* 28, no. 3 (2002): 8–9.

McFarland, Dorothy F. "District 12." *The Indiana Nurse* 29, no. 3 (1965): 36.

"Military News." *The Indiana Nurse* 29, no. 4 (1965): 21.

"Military News." *The Indiana Nurse* 31, no. 1 (1967): 20–21.

"Mr. C. D. Is Pleased to Announce." *The Indiana Nurse* 24, no. 2 (1960): 18.

Mundell, Eric. "Karren E. Mundell Vietnam Correspondence, 1966–1967 Biographical Sketch," 18 January 2003. http://www.indianahistory.org/library/manuscripts/collection_guides/m0700.html

"News." *AJN* 39, no. 11 (1939): 1,278.

"News." *AJN* 31, no. 12 (1931): 1,455.

"News About Nursing." *AJN* 40, no. 12 (1940): 1,428.

Nursing and Health Care 16, nos. 2, 4, 5 (1995) Baccalaureate, associate, and master's degree programs in nursing accredited by the NLN 1994–95.

"Nursing News and Announcements." *AJN* 21 (1921): 742.

"Official Reports of Societies—Fort Wayne, Ind." *AJN* 4, no. 4 (January 1904): 314.

"Official Reports, The Indiana Bill for the State Registration of Nurses." *AJN* 5, no. 7 (April 1905): 465–66.

"Official Reports." *AJN* 7, no. 11 (August 1907): 808.

Palmer, Sophia F. "The Effect of State Registration upon Training Schools." *AJN* 5 (1905): 657.

Parr, Suzanne, and Toby Etchels. "Serving the Profession Since 1903: A Brief History of the Indiana State Nurses' Association." *The Indiana Nurse* (1993): 63–69.

Patchin, Naomi, ed. "Commission on Economic and General Welfare." *The Indiana Nurse* (1985): 13.

_____ "Committee on Legislation." *The Indiana Nurse* (1987): 24.

_____ "Peer Review and Assistance Committee." *The Indiana Nurse* (1987): 27.

_____ "Staff Report." *The Indiana Nurse* (1987): 36.

_____ "President's Report." *ISNA Bulletin* 15, no. 6 (1989): 1 and 4.

_____ "Committee on Resolutions." *The Indiana Nurse* (1989): 47.

_____ "Peer Review and Assistance Committee." *The Indiana Nurse* (1991): 37.

_____ "108th General Assembly, First General Session." *Legislative Alert* 13, no. 6 (1993): 1.

_____ "108th General Assembly, First General Session." *Legislative Alert* 13, no. 7 (1993): 1.

_____ "President's Report." *The Indiana Nurse* (1993): 14.

_____ "ISNA-Nurse PAC." *The Indiana Nurse* (1995): 54.

_____ "Committee on Legislation." *The Indiana Nurse* (1995): 28.

_____ "ISNA-Nurse PAC." *The Indiana Nurse* (1997): 37.

_____ "Task Force on Continuing Education." *The Indiana Nurse* (1999): 50.

"President's Message." *The Indiana Nurse* 25, no. 6 (1961): 6.

"Professional Nursing." *The Indiana Nurse* 28, no. 1 (1964): 17–18.

"Professional Organization vs. Unionism, ANA Statement." *The Indiana Nurse* 27, no. 1 (1963): 22–23.

"Progress of State Registration." *AJN* 5, no. 7 (April 1905): 414.

"Progress of State Registration." *AJN* 6, no. 4 (January 1906): 213.

"Red Cross to the Rescue." *AJN* 33, no. 3 (1933): 228.

Report of the State Board of Registration and Examination of Nurses for the State of Indiana, for the Year Ending Sept. 30, 1922. Indianapolis: Wm. B. Burford, 1923.

"Resolutions Adopted by 1979 ISNA House of Delegates." *ISNA Bulletin* 5, no. 6 (1979): 3.

Scott, Elizabeth Fisher. "Public Health Nursing—On the Navajo." *The Indiana Nurse* (1956): 7–8.

Seigel, Peggy B. "She Went to War: Indiana Women Nurses in the Civil War." *Indiana Magazine of History* 86 (1990): 1–27.

Shinn, Linda, ed. "President's Report." *The Indiana Nurse* (1981): 14.

Staupers, Mabel K. "Story of the National Association of Colored Graduate Nurses." *AJN* 51, no. 4 (April 1951): 223.

Teal, Helen. "Indiana's ERA Nursing Institutes." *AJN* 34, no. 12 (December 1934): 1,158.

"The Army Needs Nurses." *The Indiana Nurse* (April 1951): 6.

"The Editor," *AJN* 1, no. 2 (November 1900): 166. *The Indiana Nurse.* April 1952. *The Lamp* 4, no. 3 (November 1940): 4.

"The President's Message." *The Indiana Nurse* 31, no. 2 (1967): 4.

"U.S. Surgeon General Endorses Nurses' Pay Drive." *The Indiana Nurse* 31, no. 1 (1967): 5.

Wall, Barbra Mann. "Grace under Pressure: The Nursing Sisters of the Holy Cross, 1861–1865." *Nursing History Review* 1 (1993): 71–87.

Wall, Lucille. "Legal Aspects of Closed Chest Cardiac Resuscitation." *The Indiana Nurse* 29, no. 4 (1965): 26.

Wood, Ann Douglas. "The War within a War: Women Nurses in the Union Army." *Civil War History* 18 (1972): 197–212.